Recognizing Brain Injury

Core Principles of Acute Neurology

Providing Acute Care
Handling Difficult Situations
Communicating Prognosis

Recognizing Brain Injury

EELCO F. M. WIJDICKS, M.D., PH.D., FACP, FNCS, FANA
Professor of Neurology, Mayo Clinic College of Medicine
Chair, Division of Critical Care Neurology
Consultant, Neurosciences Intensive Care Unit
Saint Marys Hospital
Mayo Clinic, Rochester, Minnesota

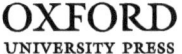

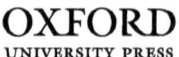

Oxford University Press is a department of the University of Oxford.
It furthers the University's objective of excellence in research, scholarship,
and education by publishing worldwide.

Oxford   New York
Auckland   Cape Town   Dar es Salaam   Hong Kong   Karachi
Kuala Lumpur   Madrid   Melbourne   Mexico City   Nairobi
New Delhi   Shanghai   Taipei   Toronto

With offices in
Argentina   Austria   Brazil   Chile   Czech Republic   France   Greece
Guatemala   Hungary   Italy   Japan   Poland   Portugal   Singapore
South Korea   Switzerland   Thailand   Turkey   Ukraine   Vietnam

Oxford is a registered trademark of Oxford University Press
in the UK and certain other countries.

Published in the United States of America by
Oxford University Press
198 Madison Avenue, New York, NY 10016

© Mayo Foundation for Medical Education and Research 2014

All rights reserved. No part of this publication may be reproduced, stored in a
retrieval system, or transmitted, in any form or by any means, without the prior
permission in writing of Oxford University Press, or as expressly permitted by law,
by license, or under terms agreed with the appropriate reproduction rights organization.
Inquiries concerning reproduction outside the scope of the above should be sent to the
Rights Department, Oxford University Press, at the address above.

You must not circulate this work in any other form
and you must impose this same condition on any acquirer.

Library of Congress Cataloging-in-Publication Data
Wijdicks, Eelco F. M., 1954– author.
Recognizing brain injury / Eelco F. M. Wijdicks.
p. ; cm. — (Core principles of acute neurology; 1)
Includes bibliographical references.
ISBN 978–0–19–992874–3 (alk. paper)
I. Title.   II. Series: Core principles of acute neurology.
[DNLM: 1. Brain Injuries. WL 354]
RC387.5
617.4′81044—dc23
2013027596

The science of medicine is a rapidly changing field. As new research and clinical experience broaden
our knowledge, changes in treatment and drug therapy occur. The author and publisher of this
work have checked with sources believed to be reliable in their efforts to provide information that
is accurate and complete, and in accordance with the standards accepted at the time of publication.
However, in light of the possibility of human error or changes in the practice of medicine, neither
the author, nor the publisher, nor any other party who has been involved in the preparation or
publication of this work warrants that the information contained herein is in every respect accurate
or complete. Readers are encouraged to confirm the information contained herein with other
reliable sources, and are strongly advised to check the product information sheet provided by the
pharmaceutical company for each drug they plan to administer.

For Barbara, Coen, and Marilou

Contents

Preface ix
Introduction to the Series xi

1. Neurology of Acute Injury 1
2. Neurology of Intracranial Pressure 17
3. Neurology of Cerebrospinal Fluid 29
4. Neurology of Unconsciousness 43
5. Neurology of Breathing 59
6. Neurology of Blood Pressure 77
7. Neurology of Cardiac Function 91
8. Neurology of Gastroenterology 105
9. Neurology of the Bladder 117
10. Troubleshooting: Localization Pearls 129

Index 145

Preface

Acute brain injury—particularly when it involves a new intracranial mass or swelling—changes the dynamics of cerebral blood flow, cerebrospinal fluid mechanics, and eventually intracranial pressure. Furthermore, acute extensive neuronal injury impacts on breathing regulation, heart function, blood pressure control, and even bowel and bladder function. It is necessary to understand not only these fundamentals but also how certain aspects of care could influence these changes in physiology. Interventions are based on current knowledge of how these systems work and interact and what happens when these systems are deregulated in the acutely ill neurologic patient.

This book is a primer—and a good deal more—on the workings of the central nervous system tailored to acute neurologic conditions. The book deals primary with acute injury to the hemispheres or brainstem but spinal cord injury is discussed where appropriate. The book ends with the basics of neurologic examination in acute brain and spine injury. What are the consequences of an acute brain injury? How does intracranial pressure relate to acute brain injury and what changes? How does the circulation of cerebrospinal fluid change? How does acute brain injury cause unconsciousness? How do we explain certain breathing patterns? How does the blood pressure influence cerebral blood flow? How does the heart become damaged, and what affects its neural control? Why does the gut stops functioning? How is bladder function affected in acute spinal cord injury?

These chapters will answer these common questions. Each of the chapters can be used not only for a comprehensive review but also to assist in care and to teach these principles.

Introduction to the Series

The confrontation with an acutely ill neurologic patient is quite an unsettling situation for physicians, but all will have to master how to manage the patient at presentation, how to shepherd the unstable patient to an intensive care unit, and how to take charge. To do that aptly, knowledge of the principles of management is needed. Books on the clinical practice of acute, emergency, and critical care neurology have appeared, but none have yet treated the fundamentals in depth.

Core Principles of Acute Neurology is a series of short volumes that handles topics not found in sufficient detail elsewhere. The books focus precisely on those areas that require a good working knowledge. These are: the consequences of acute neurologic diseases, medical care in all its aspects and relatedness with the injured brain, difficult decisions in complex situations. Because the practice involves devastatingly injured patients, there is a separate volume on prognostication and neuropalliation. Other volumes are planned in the future.

The series has unique features. I hope to contextualize basic science with clinical practice in a readable narrative with a light touch and without wielding the jargon of this field. The ten chapters in each volume try to spell out in the clearest terms how things work. The text is divided into a description of principles followed by its relevance to practice—keeping it to the bare essentials. There are boxes inserted into the text with quick reminders ("By the Way") and useful percentages carefully researched and vetted for accuracy ("By the Numbers"). Drawings are used to illustrate mechanisms and pathophysiology.

These books cannot cover an entire field, but brevity and economy allows a focus on one topic at a time. Gone are the days of large, doorstop tomes with many words on paper but with little practical value. This series is therefore characterized by simplicity—in a good sense—and it is acute and critical care neurology at the core, not encyclopedic but representative. I hope it supplements clinical curricula or comprehensive textbooks.

The audience is primarily neurologists and neurointensivists, neurosurgeons, fellows, and residents. Neurointensivists have increased in numbers, and many major institutions have attendings and fellowship programs. However, these books cross disciplines and should also be useful for intensivists, anesthesiologists, emergency physicians, nursing staff, and allied health care professionals in intensive care units and the emergency department. In the end the intent is to write a book that provides a sound reassuring basis to practice well, and that helps with understanding and appreciating the complexities of care of a patient with an acute neurologic condition.

1

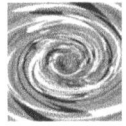

Neurology of Acute Injury

Acute injury to the brain has immediate and often prolonged damaging effects. There is a sequence of events—which is to say—there are stages of injury.[3] The brain is expressly more vulnerable to a major insult than any other tissue because its energy metabolism is high, while at the same time, it is critically dependent on aerobic metabolism of glucose and lacks sufficient capability of energy storage.[10] The energy is used not only for neuronal signaling, but also to maintain cellular machinery predominantly pumping ions across the cell membrane. In many circumstances of acute brain injury, there is a fairly simple biochemical process that results in the rapid loss of a substrate. This results in insufficient adenosine triphosphate (ATP) to keep ion pumps working, major changes in intracellular concentrations of Na^+ and K^+, membrane hyperpolarization, depolarization-facilitated Ca^+ influx, and release of the excitatory neurotransmitter glutamate, which is the primary event leading to neuronal demise, with many major neurologic insults resulting in apoptosis.[2,9]

Acute brain injury is often due to trauma, or ischemia in combination with anoxia, which surpasses causes such as acute demyelination, excitotoxicity from seizures, or destruction from infection. The long axons of neurons are predisposed to injury, but there are upstream and downstream effects that are hard to stop once injury has taken place. After the initial injury, the distal portion of the axon undergoes Wallerian degeneration: the cell body may enter an apoptotic pathway that leads to chromatolysis and swelling. Loss of synaptic boutons contacting the surface ("synaptic stripping"), phagocytosis of synapses, and replacement by microglial cells is expected soon after the injury. The molecular biology that involves interactions between receptors, signaling proteins, and cytokines is complex, and only partially resolved. Concepts on pathophysiology are constantly changing but once a neuron is lost, very little can be done because regeneration in the central nervous system is poor and disorganized.

What does this knowledge tell us about how to manage patients with acute brain injury? How much is guided by preprogrammed cascades of injury? What happens at the microscopic level, and how can we best view the effects of acute brain injury? This chapter introduces the pathophysiological mechanisms in common causes of acute brain injury. It also discusses consequences of acute brain injury that are clinically relevant and could be affected by therapeutic interventions.

Principles

Major mechanisms of acute brain injury are shown in Figure 1.1. Most of what we know about acute brain injury has been derived from tissue specimens. These neuropathologic findings are then correlated with clinical events, and, most of the time, the explanation is adequate. A clinicopathological correlation remains the mainstay of understanding the mechanism of acute neurologic injury; however, improvement in monitoring of the brain *intravitam* has shown far more changes within brain structure than is apparent from neuroimaging or electrophysiologic studies.

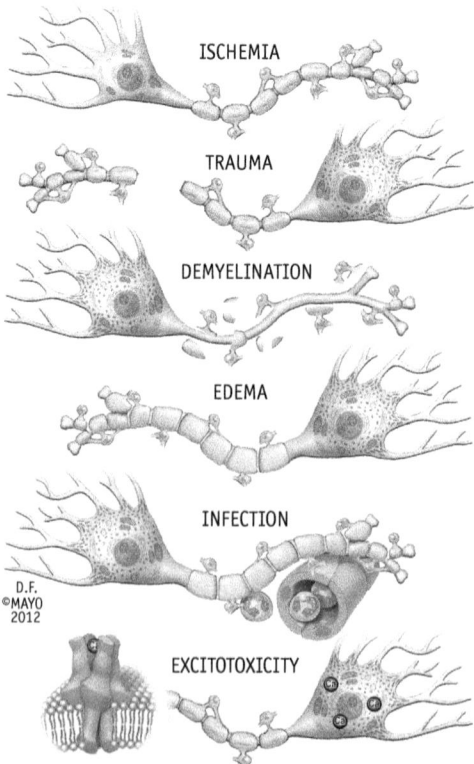

Figure 1.1 Primary mechanisms of injury to the brain.

MECHANISMS OF ACUTE BRAIN INJURY

Neuronal death can be understood as necrosis or apoptosis.[15,25] Necrosis may be far more programmed than had been previously understood—a complex enzymatic process including cytoplasmic swelling, dissolution of the cell nucleus and cell membrane apoptosis plays a major role in ischemic injury. One core principle is that there are different targets and different vulnerabilities in acute brain injury. Each major cause of brain injury is examined in this introductory chapter.

Anoxic–Ischemic Injury

Ischemia is a common cause of brain injury. It has been established that focal ischemia due to interruption of the vascular supply from hypotension (watershed areas) or occlusion by a thrombus or embolus (single vascular area) rapidly creates what are known as an ischemic core and an ischemic penumbra.[1,2] The ischemic penumbra still has intact ion pumps, normal ATP levels, and high energy metabolism, but electric activity of the neurons stops. Restoration of blood flow, however, can reverse this state. It is less clear, though, whether reperfusion of the penumbra is possible in global cerebral ischemia. This is because certain areas (hippocampal CA1 pyramidal cells), pyramidal neurons (Layers 3, 5, 6), Purkinje cells, and striatum are very vulnerable and less than 10 minutes of ischemia is enough to produce neuronal death, regardless of the restoration of blood flow.

Another common cause of acute brain injury is global diffuse ischemia after cardiac and circulatory arrest followed by resuscitation. This injury is called hypoxic-ischemic injury, but it is well known that hypoxemia or even anoxia alone rarely causes neuronal injury. During anoxia cerebral blood flow increases, hypoxemia results in hyperventilation and increased tidal volume, and hypoxemia shifts the oxygen hemoglobin curve toward more oxygen unloading. Neuronal necrosis requires ischemia which indirectly stagnates oxygen supply.

The brain has areas vulnerable to injury: in the frontal gyrus, globus pallidus, and cerebellar cortex, where Purkinje cells are located. The corpus striatum, thalamus, and pituitary gland are also predilection sites for a global ischemic insult.[15] The explanation of why certain neurons are more vulnerable than others may have to do with the number of excitatory receptors (N-methyl-D-aspartate, or NMDA; α-amino-3-hydroxy-5-methyl-4-isoxazolepropionic acid, or AMPA) and with differences in intrinsic neurophysiology. This becomes apparent in the differences seen with certain neurotoxins: CO intoxication damages the globus pallidus, while methanol intoxication damages the nearby putamen.[15]

The brainstem is resilent to ischemic injury, but if cardiopulmonary arrest is associated with a near exsanguination, or if cardiopulmonary arrest has been extremely long, the brainstem can show severe anoxic-ischemic damage. In the cortex, as expected, abnormalities are mostly in occipital-parietal areas because it is a watershed area. There is also an important watershed area between anterior and middle cerebral arteries and in the entire white matter. Whether the cortex as a whole or only watershed areas are involved depends on the insult (shock vs. cardiac arrest).

The biomechanical changes associated with ischemia and hypoxemia are complicated. Ischemia plays an important role because, as mentioned, pure hypoxemia, unless the PO_2 is very low, causes only temporary injury and rarely structural injury. When ischemia occurs, there is exposure to the excitatory neurotransmitter glutamate, which activates the NMDA receptors and AMPA receptors. This eventually leads to opening of the calcium and sodium channels. Increased calcium level will activate endonucleases that will initiate an apoptosis pathway. Increased calcium level will also accelerate lipid degradation and increase intercellular free fatty acids. The cytoskeleton proteins will also autolyze as a result of activation of calcium-dependent proteinases. This will lead to dysfunction of cellular signal and transduction systems, and axonal transport will be disturbed by dissolution of microtubules. This process will then become irreducible and final.[25]

More specifically, the ischemic cascade involves neurotransmitter receptors and excitotoxicity, inflammatory mechanisms, oxidative stress, and apoptotic mechanisms.[9,19] The blood-brain barrier (BBB) protects the brain from an inflammatory response, but when this barrier is compromised, lymphocytes gain access. Excitotoxicity is largely determined by increase of the extracellular glutamate, and there are three major glutamate receptors: NMDA, AMPA, and kainic-acid (KA). The NMDA receptor activation mediates the injury to the cerebral cortex, basal ganglia, hippocampus, and thalamus in patients with a hypoxic-ischemic insult. The AMPA receptors exacerbate the situation via sodium flux, which leads the calcium-permeable AMPA receptor channels to eventually trigger a cascade of intracellular events resulting in apoptotic pathways. Inflammatory pathways may also play a role through microglia by producing proinflammatory cytokines, and protease reactive oxygen species and complement factors may all play an important role in creating further permanent damage. In addition, excess calcium influx through glutamate receptors leads to severe excitative stress. Activation of nitrogen-oxide synthase generates reactive oxygen species. With increased reactive oxygen species levels the oxidative stress levels may result in mitochondrial permeability, uncoupling oxidative phosphorylation and resulting in mitochondrial swelling. This also activates the initial steps of apoptosis.

Apoptosis typically occurs through an extrinsic and intrinsic pathway. In the extrinsic pathway component FAS is a death receptor activated by death ligands (the ligand is FASL). This leads to caspase 8 activation and the so-called caspase cascade, and the cleaved caspase results in apoptosis. On the other hand, intrinsic pathways come within the cell and mitochondrial apoptotic signaling leads to the release of cytochrome-C, which activates caspase 9 and caspase 3. Sometimes an apoptosis inducing factor (AIF) may be released from the mitochondria, which might directly lead to activation of caspases (Figure 1.2).

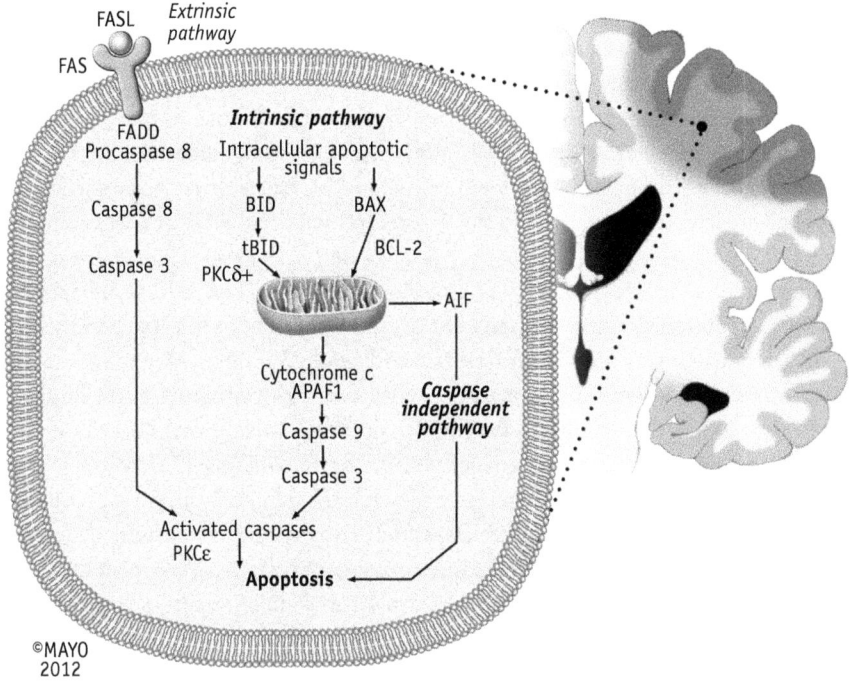

Figure 1.2 Mechanism of apoptosis.

A related cause of acute brain injury is hypoglycemia, which is often due to insulin overdose or medication error. Hypoglycemic brain injury is histologically and biochemically different from global ischemia. Hypoglycemic brain injury—in contrast to ischemic injuries—is a consequence of excess aspartate, which then causes an excitotoxic state in which lesions develop in the cerebral cortex and hippocampus (mostly CA1 dentate), though the cerebellum and brainstem are spared.

Dendritic swelling can be followed by necrosis, but no infarction takes place. In clinical practice, hypoglycemia causing persistent coma may be accompanied by hypoxemia and shock if the patient is not found until after a significant time span, and the brain injury may be a combination of these two factors.

Traumatic Brain Injury

Another very common cause of injury to the brain is traumatic brain injury (TBI). Sheared-off axons retract into globoid structures, also known as retraction balls, and rapid Wallerian degeneration is seen in the white matter and brainstem tracts.[8,21,23] Axonal injury—often the severing of multiple small axons—results in degeneration of the distal segment, causing atrophy of the white matter tracts. The axonal membrane cannot fend off calcium influx, resulting in calcium-instigated apoptosis. Most interesting is—that under experimental conditions—the process may be progressive with apoptotic mechanism remaining two weeks after injury.

Brain injury can also result in capillary damage and contusions (from punctate to small linear hemorrhages to sizable hematomas). It is well recognized that contusions may occur in a delayed fashion. Contusions can occur where bony surfaces of the skull are irregular and, thus, in the frontal and temporal areas and less common occipitally, where the skull is smooth.[15] The damage to the brain after acute subdural hematoma may also be due to compression or ischemia beneath the hematoma. Out-of-proportion swelling (without a blossoming contusion) can also occur.

Much of the injury after traumatic brain injury is through a secondary mechanism of cerebral edema. Brain swelling in adults with traumatic brain injury is often associated with multiple parenchymal contusions, shearing lesions, and traumatic subarachnoid hemorrhage. Diffuse brain swelling is also more common in children and may be a cause of subsequent deterioration in a previously alert patient. Brain edema has been classified as vasogenic edema, which is a consequence of damage to the BBB leading to increased capillary permeability, and cytotoxic edema, which is a consequence of a direct cellular insult leading to swelling without abnormalities in capillary permeability.

Alterations in ionic gradients lead eventually into cellular edema followed by vasogenic edema. Generally, cytotoxic edema is a result of intracellular accumulation of sodium. Vasogenic edema is the result of loss of integrity of the BBB.[28] Cerebral edema may be due to endothelial dysfunction and increased activity of NKCC1 transporter, upregulation of SUR1, and vasopressin receptor function. This may lead to new approaches respectively bumetanide (NKCC1 inhibitor), glibenclamide (SUR1 inhibitor), and conivaptan (vasopressin receptor antagonist).[28]

Injury from Demyelination

A less common cause of acute brain injury is acute demyelination; this has been characterized into four patterns[16]: macrophage-associated demyelination, antibody/complement-associated demyelination, distal dying back oligodendrogliopathy, and primary oligodendrocyte degeneration. The biochemical changes that occur with demyelination are an increase in water, decrease of myelin proteins, and disappearance of galactocerebroside, cholesterol-rich membranes among other complex lipids. Structural proteins such as myelin basic protein and proteolipids all decrease, and myelin is replaced by extracellular fluid, astrocytes, and inflammatory cells. Microscopic examination of brain tissue shows loss of myelin but preservation of axons, predominant T-lymphocyte infiltrates also consisting of macrophages and microglia. However, most concerning is a more fulminant form of acute demyelination with rapid progression and inflammatory demyelinating lesions. Such a lesion may become a mass (Marburg disease) or diffusely spread throughout the white matter (acute disseminated encephalomyelitis). When the lesion is biopsied, lymphocytes are commonly seen in early lesions.

Injury from Infection

Central nervous system infections can also cause an acute rapid injury of the neuronal integrity. The mechanism, however, is far more complex and involves changes in the BBB and immune activation. Bacteria do not enter easily and have to overcome the BBB, but once they pass through, they multiply rapidly in cerebrospinal fluid (CSF) and incite an inflammatory response. The rapid inflammatory response is likely a result of released bacterial products.[18] Moreover, certain bacteria can activate plasminogen, resulting in damage of the intracellular matrix and basement membrane of the BBB. Cytokines—including tumor necrosis factor and interleukins—are released, and levels remain high, which activates complement and clotting cascades. The injury here might be caused by abscess formation, cortical necrosis, and a combination of cytogenic, vasogenic, and interstitial edema. Brain edema is initially a reflection of increased blood-brain permeability, but abnormal CSF outflow to the venous system (Chapter 3) from high resistance in the arachnoid villi contributes later. The toxins associated with bacterial infection of the central nervous system are likely responsible for the initiation of the caspase apoptosis pathways.[18] Coagulation abnormalities may also play an important role in the development of a secondary injury to the brain through a cerebral intravascular coagulopathy. Cerebral blood flow is also an important component, with a marked decrease due to vasospasm and vasculitis. All these above-mentioned injury mechanisms are in full force before the first dose of antibiotics, and in fact destruction of the bacterial cell wall may release products that further increase the proinflammatory cytokines.

Injury from Excitotoxicity and Toxins

Finally, seizures can damage the brain. Seizures can be seen as a result of a dysbalance between neuronal inhibition and excitation. It has always been best understood as neuronal cells use more energy, following which sodium and calcium can enter the cell during persistent seizures, resulting in enhanced excitability.[12] Hippocampal neuronal injury is also prominent here. Excitatory amino acids are also implicated in injury associated with epilepsy. There is a reduction of gamma-aminobutyric acid (GABA) and increase in NMDA and AMPA glutamate receptors.

A more complex understanding of acute brain injury includes consideration of neurotoxins in some cases of neurotoxicity and this occurs through the mechanism of cerebral edema. This is particularly likely in acute fulminant hepatic failure, in which increased ammonia causes postsynaptic inhibition in the cortex, thalamus, and brainstem and also decreases glutamatergic synaptic function. Cerebral edema may occur in acute liver necrosis from drug intoxication (mostly acetaminophen), and a multifold increase in glutamine has been implicated. Glutamine is an osmolyte and increases brain water. Swelling of the astrocyte may also result in production of reactive oxygen and nitrogen oxygen species that, in itself, may cause vasodilatation and hyperemia, and may further increase cerebral edema and intracranial pressure. Again, here the mechanism is likely apoptosis as a result of the in ability of glial cells to overcome the osmotic challenge.

SECONDARY INSULTS AFTER ACUTE BRAIN INJURY

Another core principle of acute brain injury is that each of these abnormalities can cause secondary injuries through the mechanism of brain displacement (Figure 1.3). Brain swelling displaces brain tissue and secondarily results in compression of the diencephalic structures and injury to the brainstem. Therefore, care of acutely ill neurologic patients is often not just the treatment of the initial injury but also prevention of a secondary injury (Figure 1.3). Some patients, by the nature of their injury, may have a certain expected outcome that can become markedly different if an additional injury occurs. There is a potential, even if intermittently brief of damaging effects of hypoxemia, hypotension, anemia,

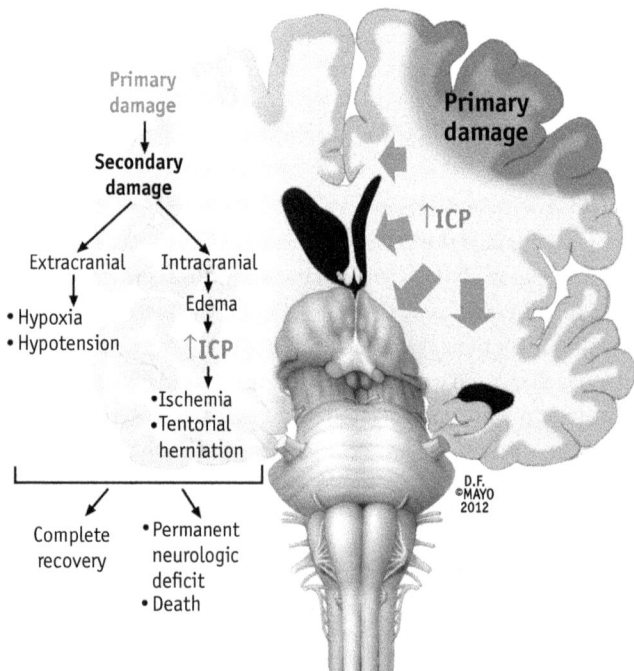

Figure 1.3 Mechanism of secondary brain injury.

and possibly hypercarbia. As mentioned before, brain edema can be due to a vasogenic mechanism or a cytotoxic mechanism, but often a combination of both occurs. In vasogenic edema, the breakdown of the BBB results in swollen myelin sheaths and, later, swollen astrocytes and thus this will further result in more mass, less space and no place to go other than through the tentorium

Uncontrolled ICP or severe secondary injury may lead to permanent total brain stem dysfunction. This outcome however remains uncommon occurring in less than 10% of catastrophic injuries. If every possible confounder has been excluded, irreversible loss of brain function is clinically recognized as the absence of brainstem reflexes, verified apnea, loss of vascular tone, invariant heart rate, and, eventually, cardiac standstill. This condition cannot be reversed—not even partly—by medical or surgical intervention, and is fundamentally absolute. It is an acceptable neurologic definition of death. A need to demonstrate loss of all neuronal function through absence of intracranial circulation or absence of electrical activity would remain—for a substantial minority of physicians, including neurologists and neurosurgeons—the only proof of brain death.

The neuropathologic findings are markedly variable, and many areas of the brain do not seem affected despite permanent loss of brain function. Even a state of no blood flow to the brain, using current cerebral blood flow studies, does not lead to a complete liquefied brain, and thus identifiable structures remain when examined pathologically following weeks of—albeit notoriously difficult ventilatory and circulatory support—support.

In Practice

Once confronted with a patient with an acute brain injury, three questions remain: First, how can we monitor the patient? Second, how can we intervene? and third how does this ultimately help to the patient? Neurosciences intensive care units will have to rely on repeated expert neurologic examination, neuroimaging and electrophysiology to ensure that acute brain injury does not worsen.

MONITORING ACUTE BRAIN INJURY

Brain function can currently be monitored using parameters such as intracranial pressure (ICP), brain tissue oxygenation, and microdialysis, each of which may signal neuronal distress. Electroencephalography (EEG)-video monitoring may be used in patients with a fluctuating level of consciousness after a single seizure and to titrate antiepileptic drugs.

One of the most demanding issues in the care of an acutely injured neurologic patient is to find a reliable device or probe that can monitor brain dysfunction continuously. Real-time assessment of global or regional brain dysfunction could help clinicians recognize early worsening, prompt specific management changes, and monitor response to therapy. Monitoring devices are most useful in sedated and paralyzed patients, when neurologic examination is limited to the assessment of pupillary size and light reflex. In all other cases, the findings from any monitoring device need to be seen as complementing a detailed and comprehensive clinical neurologic examination. Cerebral monitoring devices can provide a wealth of physiological information, but it remains to be seen if treatment guided by such information can improve clinical outcomes. Recent history has taught us that the use of even some of the most uniformly accepted devices may fail to improve clinical outcome—we are reminded of the pulmonary artery catheter saga.

If one device does not do it all, then why not use more than one device? Thus the term "multimodality" (referring to multiple modes of input) has come into vogue. Multimodality monitoring in the neurosciences intensive care unit can involve monitoring of ICP, microdialysis, brain tissue oxygenation, near-infrared spectroscopy, and digital EEG with quantitative analysis, often all at the same time. Crucial questions remain as to whether the monitored events require an intervention and what should be the thresholds to intervene.

The potential usefulness of continuous EEG monitoring in the intensive care unit has been recently demonstrated. Continuous EEG is an expensive and labor-intensive program and requires expertise for interpretation. However, it has been shown that in many comatose patients, seizures are not clinically recognized, and this applies to both convulsive and nonconvulsive seizures. EEG may have a role in the detection of cerebral ischemia after subarachnoid hemorrhage and may also help detect episodes of cortical spreading depression, which can affect the control of ICP or blood pressure.

These and other techniques hold promise and need to be studied carefully in separate cohorts of patients. We know that findings from various monitoring modalities can refine our clinical assessment, but we still need to find out if they can guide therapy to improve clinical outcome. Novel noninvasive devices will likely become available in the near future. None of the current methods have been hailed as the ultimate way of monitoring, so this approach would likely require a new original way. Multimodal brain monitoring does allow information gathering that is otherwise not available, and noninvasive approaches are now a focus of development. Proponents of such an approach have not resolved the major pitfalls of these systems: unknown significance, unknown interobserver variability, unknown thresholds for intervention, unknown effect on outcome.

Brain monitoring has been synonymous with ICP monitoring as a technique for observing the brain for many years (and still is in many places). Another example is brain tissue oximetry, which recognizes changes in brain oxygenation. The concept is that oxygen levels decrease when neurons are at risk of ischemia; and therefore, brain oxygen pressure could be related to cerebral blood flow. Studies have found not only that patients with low brain tissue oxygen values are at higher risk of a poor outcome but also that outcome can be improved with treatment of these values by increasing systemic oxygenation or cerebral perfusion pressure.

Others have defined a neurometabolic crisis as a low glucose concentration or elevation in the lactate to pyruvate ratio.[13,17,24] Temporal patterns of abnormal lactate to pyruvate ratios were associated with increased mortality and unfavorable outcome independent of ICP, Glasgow coma scale, or age. The main question remains whether these findings on microdialysis represent an early indication of irreversible brain damage or provide an opportunity for intervention. The assumption here is that lactate and pyruvate levels reflect neuronal ischemia. Using cerebral microdialysis probes, glucose, lactate, and pyruvate can be measured, and the duration of "metabolic crisis" may predict outcome or tissue loss after a major injury.

Another way of evaluating neuronal distress is to evaluate patients for the appearance of spreading depolarization.[4,5,6,7,11,26] The basic premise behind this concept is that spreading depolarization of neurons reflects breakdown of ion gradients. Mostly the sodium and calcium pumps provide insufficient outward current to balance the inward current of sodium and potassium, leading to inactivation of action potentials at the membrane channels. During spreading depolarization, neuronal signaling is markedly depressed and this mechanism may play a role in anoxic-ischemic injury, hypoglycemia, stroke, subarachnoid hemorrhage, status epilepticus, or TBI.[11,27,19] Spreading depolarization can only be detected using subdural electrodes providing an electrocorticography and, therefore, only can be monitored in selected patients. It is assumed that these repetitive spreading depolarizations are indicative of neuronal injury and could also be used to monitor the development of cerebral ischemia. When this depolarization occurs, the circulation either becomes hyperdynamic or hypodynamic, which may further progress the ischemia and neuronal distress; hence, the spreading of depolarization.

There is major research interest in finding a reliable biomarker of acute brain injury in serum and CSF, just as biomarkers can be diagnostic, predictive, or both in the fields of oncology, acute cardiovascular disease, and autoimmune diseases. The type of injury may result in biomarkers specific to the acute brain injury. The value of these biomarkers (single or a panel) remains to be established, but they could become independent predictors of a certain clinical course (e.g., developing cerebral edema) and outcome (markers of severity of injury and potential for recovery). To illustrate this further, for example, the early events of the ischemic cascade, including glial activation, result in release of biomarkers that are relatively specific to glial function: S100B, glial fibrillary acidic protein, and myelin basic protein. Any component of the ischemic cascade may be investigated and may include lipid peroxidation, inflammatory, and endothelial dysfunction. In TBI and anoxic ischemic injury neuron-specific enolase (NSE) have been studied but with variable predictive value. Other possibly meaningful CSF biomarkers are glial fibrillary acidic protein (GFAP), ubiquitin C-terminal hydrolase-L1 (UCH-L1), and αII-spectrin breakdown product (SBDP).[14]

The integrity of the BBB is important and may predict the development of cerebral edema or hemorrhagic conversion. Matrix metalloproteinase-9 (a major BBB-degrading enzyme) and cellular fibronectin (a constituent of the basal lamina) have been associated with later clinically significant cerebral edema.

INTERVENTION OF ACUTE BRAIN INJURY

How do we best approach acute brain injury in practice? Is this approach disease specific? One could convincingly argue that an early, very aggressive approach is warranted and trying every means to treat the problem, but that one should hold back when there is no success. Some brain injuries cannot be treated, no matter what you do. Some patients will improve beyond a devastating disability.

Many disorders can worsen; in such cases, the goal is to prevent the progression from happening. In clinical practice, it is important to determine which patient is at risk for further injury and, in particular, in which patients we can predict brain edema causing shifts and compression effects.

Brain edema develops rapidly in certain conditions, such as TBI, acute bacterial meningitis, or fulminant hepatic necrosis. Computed tomography (CT) scanning in these circumstances will demonstrate generalized edema with cortical effacement and obliteration of the basal cistern. The ventricles collapse, and displacement of major brain structures can be seen.

Brain edema can also be protracted, as in a patient with a hemispheric mass.[22] An acute cerebral infarct may take many hours to become edematous, and clinical deterioration can spread over many hours, even days. Brain edema after intracranial hemorrhage is mostly inconsequential, and the shift of brain structures is largely determined by enlargement of the hematoma and not so much the perilesional edema. However, delayed significant edema may recur and cause deterioration after a relatively unchanged time interval.

There should also be a major effort to reduce the potential damaging effects of systemic triggers such as marked hypoxemia, marked hypercarbia, or hypotension. In patients with traumatic brain injury, other trauma may cause this instability, but in other patients a procedure (e.g., bronchoscopy) that requires the use of anesthetic drugs (i.e., a propofol bolus) can all precipitate a marked hypotension. Hypotension can also occur in patients who develop a

Table 1.1 **Initial Considerations in Acute Brain Injury**

• Obtain venous and arterial access
• Avoid hypoosmolar fluids (no lactated Ringer's solution) or glucose-containing fluids (no D5W, no 0.45% NaCl)
• Avoid long-lasting sedatives
• Treat fever
• Aim for mild hypocapnia, mild hyperoxemia
• Avoid high PEEP (<10 mm Hg) to reduce intrathoracic pressure
• Consider ICP monitor
• Consider CSF drainage
• Consider neurophysiologic studies (EEG monitoring)
• Treat seizures with IV antiepileptic drugs
• Aim for hyperosmolarity (~285 mOsm/kg) with mannitol
• Consider corticosteroids (if mass)
• Consider broad-spectrum antibiotics and antivirals (if fever)

PEEP, positive end expiratory pressure; EEG, electroencephalography; ICP, intracranial pressure; CSF, cerebrospinal fluid.

nosocomial infection that evolves into sepsis. Sedation also carries the risk of hypoxemia, and hypercapnia due to upper airway obstruction. Simple procedures such as a tracheostomy could cause a sudden change in blood pressure or oxygenation that may tip the patient—already in a delicate balance—over the edge. It is not uncommon to see that the patient has a further deterioration after this procedure and with no improvement even after the inciting trigger has been treated. Seizures should be recognized, not underestimated, rapidly treated, and kept under control. There are some general clinical strategies that apply to every patient with an acute brain injury, and they are summarized in Table 1.1.

Putting It All Together

- There is marked selective vulnerability of neurons
- Acute brain injury is followed by a secondary biochemical wave of injury
- Brain edema is common after acute brain injury and determines outcome
- Brain injury may cause increased intracranial pressure and permanent injury from impaired intracranial blood flow
- Treatment of secondary insults are equally important as treatment of primary insults to the brain.

> **BY THE WAY**
>
> - Severe neuronal injury results in apoptosis
> - ICP control reduces brain injury
> - Spreading depression may be a valid mechanism of brain injury
> - Most technology to monitor the brain is expensive
> - Biomarkers could help clinicians in the future

> **ACUTE BRAIN INJURY BY THE NUMBERS**
>
> - ~ 90% of ATP production is reduced during global ischemia
> - ~ 40% of brain energy is needed to simply maintain cell integrity
> - ~ 30% of astrocytes have glycolytic capacity and produce ATP
> - ~ 20% of oxygen needed by the body goes to the brain
> - ~ 10% of brain injury is irreversible

References

1. Attwell D, Buchan AM, Charpak S, et al. Glial and neuronal control of brain blood flow. *Nature* 2010;468:232–243.
2. Dirnagl U. Pathobiology of injury after stroke: the neurovascular unit and beyond. *Ann NY Acad Sci* 2012;1268:21–25.
3. Doberstein CE, Hovda DA, Becker DP. Clinical considerations in the reduction of secondary brain injury. *Ann Emerg Med* 1993;22:993–997.
4. Dohmen C, Sakowitz OW, Fabricius M, et al. Spreading depolarizations occur in human ischemic stroke with high incidence. *Ann Neurol* 2008;63:720–728.
5. Dreier JP, Woitzik J, Fabricius M, et al. Delayed ischemic neurological deficits after sub-arachnoid hemorrhage are associated with clusters of spreading depolarizations. *Brain* 2006;129:3224–3237.
6. Dreier JP. The role of spreading depression, spreading depolarization and spreading ischemia in neurological disease. *Nat Med* 2011;17:439–447.
7. Fabricius M, Fuhr S, Bhatia R, et al. Cortical spreading depression and peri-infarct depolarization in acutely injured human cerebral cortex. *Brain* 2006;129:778–790.
8. Farkas O, Lifshitz J, Povlishock JT. Mechanoporation induced by diffuse traumatic brain injury: an irreversible or reversible response to injury? *J Neurosci* 2006;26:3130–3140.
9. Green DR, Reed JC. Mitochondria and apoptosis. *Science* 1998;281:1309–1312.
10. Harris JJ, Jolivet R, Attwell D. Sunpatic energy use and supply. *Neuron* 2012;75:762–777.
11. Hartings JA, Strong AJ, Fabricius M, et al. Spreading depolarizations and late secondary insults after traumatic brain injury. *J Neurotrauma* 2009;26:1857–1866.
12. Holmes GL. Seizure-induced neuronal injury: animal data. *Neurology* 2002;59:S3–6.
13. Lakshmanan R, Loo JA, Drake T, et al. Metabolic crisis after traumatic brain injury is associated with a novel microdialysis proteome. *Neurocrit Care* 2010;12:324–336.
14. Le Li J, Li XY, Feng DF, Pan DC. Biomarkers associated with diffuse traumatic axonal injury: exploring pathogenesis, early diagnosis, and prognosis. *J Trauma* 2010;69:1610–1618.
15. Love S, Louis DN, Ellison DW. *Greenfield's Neuropathology* 8th ed. London, Hodder Arnold, 2008.

16. Lucchinetti CF, Parisi J, Bruck W. The pathology of multiple sclerosis. *Neurol Clin* 2005;23: 77–105.
17. Marcoux J, McArthur DA, Miller C, et al. Persistent metabolic crisis as measured by elevated cerebral microdialysis lactate-pyruvate ratio predicts chronic frontal lobe brain atrophy after traumatic brain injury. *Crit Care Med* 2008;36:2871–2877.
18. Mook-Kanamori BB, Geldhoff M, van der Poll T, van de Beek D. Pathogenesis and pathophysiology of pneumococcal meningitis. *Clin Microbiol Rev* 2011;24:557–591.
19. Prineas JW, Parratt JD. Oligodendrocytes and the early multiple sclerosis lesion. *Ann Neurol* 2012;72:18–31.
20. Raghupathi R. Cell death mechanisms following traumatic brain injury. *Brain Pathol* 2004;14:215–222.
21. Shrey DW, Griesbach GS, Giza CC. The pathophysiology of concussions in youth. *Phys Med Rehabil Clin N Am* 2011;22:577–602.
22. Simard JM, Kent TA, Chen M, Tarasov KV, Gerzanich V. Brain edema in focal ischemia: molecular pathophysiology and theoretical implications. *Lancet Neurol* 2007;6:258–268.
23. Smith C. The long-term consequences of microglial activation following acute traumatic brain injury. *Neuropathol Appl Neurobiol* 2013;39:35–44.
24. Stein NR, McArthur DL, Etchepare M, Vespa PM. Early cerebral metabolic crisis after TBI influences outcome despite adequate hemodynamic resuscitation. *Neurocrit Care* 2012;17:49–57.
25. Stevens JB, Abdallah BY, Liu G, et al. Heterogeneity of cell death. *Cytogenet Genome Res* 2013;139:164–173.
26. Strong AJ, Anderson PJ, Watts HR, et al. Peri-infarct depolarizations lead to loss of perfusion in ischemic gyrencephalic cerebral cortex. *Brain* 2007;130:995–1008.
27. Strong AJ, Fabricius M, Boutelle MG, et al. Spreading and synchronous depressions of cortical activity in acutely injured human brain. *Stroke* 2002;33:2738–2743.
28. Walcott BP, Kahle KT, Simard JM. Novel treatment targets for cerebral edema. *Neurotherapeutics* 2012;9:65–72.

2

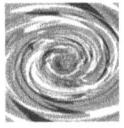

Neurology of Intracranial Pressure

Intracranial pressure (ICP) is a reflection of the total intracranial volume. The sum of its components (blood, brain, and cerebrospinal fluid) is constant but not static. One possible consequence of acute brain injury is an increase in brain volume from mass effect and simultaneous pressure increase that may occur rapidly simply because of the presence of separate compartments and a cranium. Such pressure may move brain tissue out of its own compartment and may stagnate intracranial entry of arterial blood, thus changing cerebral blood flow and eventually causing ischemia. Increased intracranial pressure under any circumstances requires immediate management if permanent damage is to be avoided, as ICP may cause brain tissue compression and brainstem shift. One of the most important principles is that increased ICP will cause brainstem injury. Brainstem injury might be the point of no return, markedly reducing the chance of recovery. Eventually brainstem injury will progress to loss of all brainstem function, clinically seen as brainstem areflexia, apnea, and hypotension, and this change is definitive. Massively increased ICP is the most common mechanism of brain death.

For physicians, clinically recognizing increased ICP may not seem difficult. It is usually judged on the basis of a CT scan (showing cerebral edema or mass effect), clinical appearance of loss of brainstem reflexes due to shift (resulting in fixed dilated or anisocoric pupils), and systemic manifestations (appearance of the Cushing reflex with increase in pulse pressure often associated with bradycardia). In many patients increased ICP cannot be inferred and only direct measurement of pressure provides the answer.

Management of increased ICP is a complicated trial-and-error exercise. It starts in the emergency room the moment the patient arrives. Any manipulation in blood pressure, oxygenation, acid/base balance, fluid administration, or drug administration can change ICP and rapidly change the relationship between pressure and volume within the skull. One observation is clear: sustained increased intracranial pressure results in higher mortality rates. Conversely, rapid reduction of increased ICP through medical therapy, cerebrospinal (CSF) diversion with a ventriculostomy or more definitive removal of a mass or a large skull fragment may reduce mortality and likely also morbidity from secondary injury.[14,22,33]

There is still little known about accurately quantifying the parameters that allow for best management. ICP monitoring provides a number followed by a calculated cerebral perfusion pressure (CPP), but this is only part of the complex picture.

For practitioners several questions remain: How can we best understand increased ICP and what causes it? What treatment for increased ICP should be tried, and when do we proceed with more urgent matters such as neurosurgical decompression? This chapter will discuss the current concepts and management of increased intracranial pressure.

Principles

Any discussion of intracranial pressure should begin with the skull. Most living species have no skulls, and vertebrates are not even 1% of all species on earth, but the skull is there to protect the brain. The skull is somewhat "flexible" early in life but later becomes rigid and does not allow acute increase in brain pressure.

It is important to sketch out some core fundamentals in understanding volume and pressure within the skull and craniospinal axis. Four compartments determine the total volume encompassed by a nonexpandable skull, and that volume is constant. This is known as the Monro-Kellie doctrine.[34] These compartments contain the venous and arterial volumes (both 5%), CSF (10%), and brain parenchyma (80%). CSF and intracranial blood volume both measure 75 mL. CSF pressure is equal throughout the CSF pathways but only if CSF flow is not obstructed somewhere.[1,2] The doctrine states that change (increase or decrease) in one compartment should be followed by a change (increase or decrease) in one or two other compartments. Usually, up to 150 mL of new volume can be compensated, but this depends on the volume of the brain parenchyma.[7,24] The normal intracranial pressure is between 0 and 10 mm Hg with a variable upper limit that is somewhere between 15 and 20 mm Hg.

What can be said about increased ICP? Neurosurgeon Douglas Miller defined three patterns:

1. Sustained high pressure. These waves—called plateau waves for their configuration—are associated with vascular dilatation and increase in cerebral blood volume without increase in cerebral blood flow.
2. Steady rise to severe intracranial hypertension >50 mm Hg.
3. Episodic waves of ICP.

In monitoring experiments, neurosurgeon Lundberg called these pressure waves A, B, and C waves.[18] Sustained elevations of ICP (>50 mm Hg) for 5–20 minutes with rapid decline were called A waves (same as the plateau waves). Brief peaks of

ICP (sometimes 1 or 2 peaks per minute) were called B waves and often occurred during Cheyne-Stokes respiration. C waves (4–8 waves per minute) were said to correspond to variations in arterial blood pressure (transient oscillations of blood pressure associated with hemodynamic changes).[19]

Whether increased ICP is clinically consequential (causing coma and associated neurologic signs) depends on the volume of the mass lesion but also the rate of expansion, the relative volume of blood and CSF, and perhaps also the anatomical configuration of the tentorial hiatus, where tissue may go if under pressure. Increased ICP may occur from an increase in volume of the CSF compartment, which causes acute hydrocephalus. More problematic is an increase of ICP when there is an increase in cerebral blood volume, which often results from arterial vasodilatation or obstruction of the venous outflow from the intracranial cavity. The most important trigger of increased cerebral blood volume from vaso dilatation is hypercarbia, which can be caused by acute pulmonary disease such as aspiration or may simply be part of the vicious cycle that is caused by decreased level of consciousness, decreased respiratory drive, and CO_2 retention. Conversely, hypocapnia and hyperoxia reduce ICP by cerebral vasoconstriction and reduction in cerebral blood volume. A similar mechanism occurs with inducing hypothermia.

The compensatory reserve, compliance, and its reverse, elastance, all measure how the brain lessens the impact of extra volume. The pressure/volume curve is in essence a curvilinear relationship but also an exponential part with rapid steepening pressure increase when these compensatory mechanisms fail.[17, 21] The basic principle is that when ICP rises, similar increments of volume (ΔV) cause larger rises of intracranial pressure (ΔP). Intracranial elastance is understood as $\Delta P/ \Delta V$ (Figure 2.1). ICP is possibly the sum of ICP due to cerebral blood volume and ICP due to CSF pressure. On the other hand, ICP is determined by the resistance in CSF outflow, CSF formation and pressure in the sagittal venous sinus. Thus, any factor that would cause obstruction of the CSF pathway would hamper the circulation and result in increased ICP.

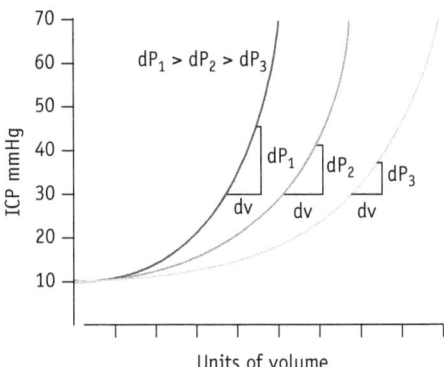

Figure 2.1 ICP-Volume relationships.

The pressure/volume curve is variable and dependent on at least three factors. First, the curve may change in the presence of a craniotomy site and brain atrophy (generalized or prior encephalomalacia) exists. Second, there is evidence that osmotic diuretics flatten the shape of the volume/pressure curve and that the brain is more tolerant of additional volume. Third, tightness of the brain is also influenced by the level of arterial blood pressure (Fig 2.1). When ICP is increased, the volume/pressure response can increase with arterial hypertension and also decrease by hypotension. Cerebral blood flow does not have any influence on the configuration of the pressure/volume curve.[16,19,22,25] Cerebral blood flow is constant despite increase in ICP, up to 30 mm Hg. However, cerebral blood flow also is constant until the difference between arterial pressure and ICP falls below 40 mm Hg. At that stage, ICP is similar to arterial transmural pressure.

There are two major types of autoregulation: pressure and metabolic autoregulation. Pressure autoregulation implies that, over a certain range of CPP, the cerebral blood flow remains constant, usually between 50 and 150 mm Hg. The main physiologic mechanism is a change in the arterial wall diameter—so, low perfusion pressure, vasodilation, high perfusion pressure, vasoconstriction. When maximally dilated, arterial walls may collapse. When maximally constricted, they may leak after they become dilated again. (For additional discussion and explanatory drawing see Chapter 6).

Typically ICP is part of the CPP formula, defined as CPP = MAP - ICP. Because CPP represents the pressure gradient across the cerebral vascular bed, it regulates cerebral blood flow and is autoregulated. The cerebral vessels need to be reactive so that an increase in CPP does not result in hyperemia, increase in vasogenic edema, and further increase in ICP.

Cerebral blood flow remains constant during rising ICP, but only when autoregulation remains intact.[3] Autoregulation disappears early in brain compression, and the CO_2 response is also lost (known as cerebral vasomotor paralysis). This limits the effect of hyperventilation, because hyperventilation works through vasomotor responsiveness. Increase in arterial pressure in patients with increased ICP may not produce an increase in cerebral blood flow but rather increase in ICP (known as false autoregulation). Blood flow does not change because ICP rises with arterial pressure; there is no change in the arterial transmural pressure or CPP and, therefore, no reason for flow to change. A similar process can occur with the so-called no-reflow phenomenon, which is failure of the brain to reperfuse after complete cardiac standstill. Cerebral blood flow cannot be reestablished because capillary wall swelling has obstructed flow.

Metabolic autoregulation implies that cerebral blood flow equals cerebral metabolism rate of oxygen ($CMRO_2$). This is best illustrated by the Fick equation $CMRO_2 = CBF \times AVDO_2$. The arteriovenous difference of O_2 ($AVDO_2$) is the jugular venous oxygen content subtracted from the arterial oxygen content. The autoregulation here is to guarantee oxygen delivery. Therefore, with poor cerebral blood flow the oxygen extraction rate increases.

Intracranial pressure can be monitored after inserting a parenchymal or ventricular sensor. The resulting waveform consists of three components and most resembles an arterial waveform because the first and fastest component is a result of the arterial pulse. The second component is from respiration (or CSF pulsations) followed by a slow wave. The ICP waveform is usually displayed in rapid chart speed. When displayed this way, three upstrokes can be identified. The first wave (WP) is the percussion wave, representing pulsation of large arteries; the second wave (WT) is the tidal wave, representing intracranial compliance; and the third wave (WD) is the dicrotic wave, representing aortic valve closure. When ICP increases, the WT becomes higher than the WP (Figure 2.2). Further analysis of the ICP waveform may reveal changes in the waveform characteristics that may reflect abnormal regulatory systems.[8]

There are basically two ways to assess the physiologic consequences of intracranial pressure increase, and both have been studied recently. The pressure-volume compensatory reserve (introduced by Lofgren and Zwetnow) is mathematically summarized by the RAP index (correlation coefficient [R] between the amplitude of the fundamental component [A] and mean pressure [P]). When the RAP index or coefficient is 0, there is no correlation between amplitude of the fundamental component of the ICP wave and the mean ICP, meaning a good pressure volume reserve—change in volume does not reflect change in pressure.[17]

With an increase of RAP to +1, there is a correlation between ICP and the fundamental component of the ICP wave indicating a place on the steep slope of the curve and compensatory reserve at risk. When the RAP declines and becomes negative (RAP < 0), there is no further cerebral autoregulation and arterioles are maximally dilated. With plateau waves, this index also decreases as a result of maximal vasodilation.

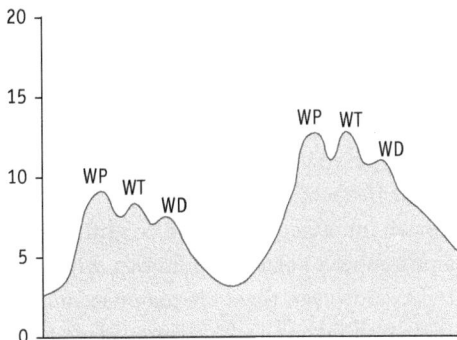

Figure 2.2 ICP waveforms and changing with increasing ICP. WP = percussion wave representing arterial pressure and transmitted at systole, WT = tidal wave representing relative brain volume or compliance increases with expanding masses and becomes higher than WP with increasing ICP. WD = dicrotic wave representing venous pulsation and aortic closure.

Another derived index is the pressure reactivity index (PRx). This index mathematically constructs the response of ICP to changes in arteriole pressure. Normally, increased blood pressure reduces cerebral volume and reduces ICP. When this reactivity is impaired, there is a passive transmission of blood pressure to ICP. A positive PRx means a passive nonreactive cerebrovascular bed. A negative value represents a normal reactive vascular bed. This index correlates well with other measures such as transcranial Doppler ultrasound, and brain microdialysis.[5,6,7,8] All these measures require sophisticated computer software, none of which is yet widely used.

Another core principle is to understand the consequences of massively increased ICP. When ICP is increased, it can lead to permanent damage through several mechanisms. The main mechanism is displacement of the thalamus-brainstem complex downward, sideways, or a combination of both, leading to progressive loss of function of this structure. Displacement of the brainstem may be a result of diffuse brain edema, or it may be caused by a single mass compressing this structure. Buckling of the brainstem leads to a sequential loss of its function, but reflexes may be lost very rapidly and all together. Damage of the pons alters the breathing drive, and breathing stops when the medulla oblongata becomes involved. Simultaneously, with involvement of the brainstem, the vagal cardiomotor centers stop providing parasympathetic activity. Unopposed vagal output leads to sympathetic stimulation and a hypertensive response.

At the same time, intracranial pressure rises substantially and seriously reduces or causes stagnation of cerebral perfusion, leading to virtual intracranial standstill and finally global profound ischemia.[27] One would expect this to occur with CPPs in the range of 10–20 mm Hg. Brain perfusion due to collapsed arterioles is nonexistent with these critical CPPs, resulting in reverberating, ineffective blood flow. Once cerebral blood flow stops in an apneic patient with completely absent brainstem reflexes, cerebral blood flow cannot return because of permanent vascular collapse, and brainstem function has never returned clinically.

Another core principle is to understand how medical management of intracranial hypertension works. Physicians have noted that using osmotic diuretics or hyperventilation allows the intracranial pressure to be reduced substantially and very quickly. Acute hyperventilation causes acute CSF alkalosis, and cerebral vasoconstriction reduces intracranial blood volume; thus, this compartment is able to compensate for an increase in pressure. Within a matter of minutes, this effect is seen. The same applies to osmotic diuretics, which draw water out of the neurons into the arteries. However, there are major secondary consequences that lead to a response. Increased intravascular volume leads to vasoconstriction and reduced cerebrovascular volume. Increased cerebral blood flow leads to reduced viscosity and increased oxygen delivery, causing vasoconstriction to normalize oxygen delivery and, consequently, reduction of ICP through reduced cerebrovascular volume[19,30] (Figure 2.3). Therefore, diuresis is not the mechanism by which ICP is reduced. It is the autoregulation of the vasculature suddenly exposed to

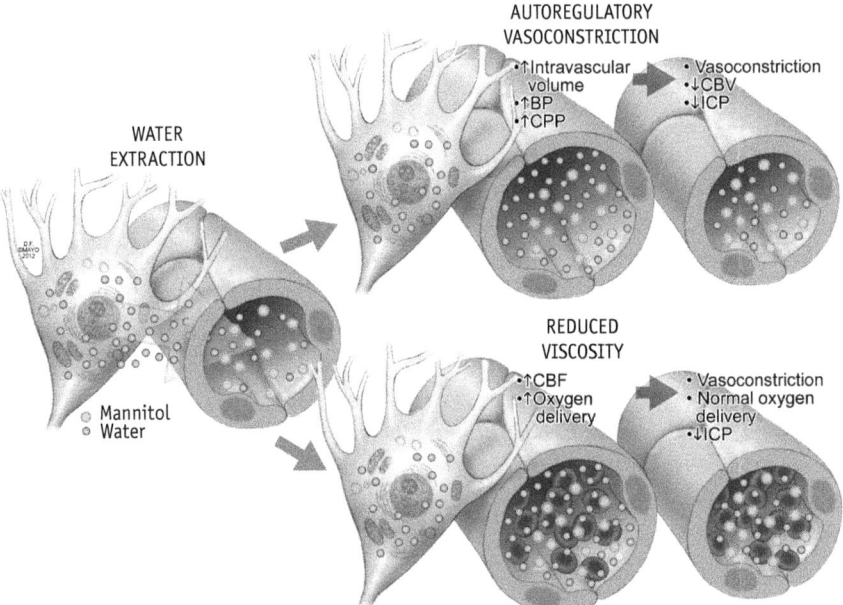

Figure 2.3 How mannitol works.

more water. Osmotic agents work through an osmotic gradient; thus, one can expect similar effects with mannitol or hypertonic saline as long as they have an osmotically equivalent dose. Hypertonic saline, therefore, does not necessarily outperform mannitol.[10-15,20,25,27]

Short-term ICP control for treating neurosurgical patients is better with infusing hypertonic saline irrespective of concentration, bolus, or continuous drip. The concentrations used are 7% to 23.4% with small volumes.[26] Hypertonic saline also reduces endothelial cell edema in the microcirculation, lowers the flow resistance, and improves cerebrovascular flow. Hypertonic saline does not produce the significant diuresis (the so-called second-pass effect) of mannitol. Hypertonic saline may act better as a volume expander in the long run, since mannitol may reduce circulating volume through diuresis later. Higher serum sodium values are also better tolerated with hypertonic saline simply because it is due to sodium surplus and not water deficit as with mannitol.[16]

In Practice

There is a complete lack of standardization of ICP monitoring and a recent survey found major differences in recording ICP values, leveling and zeroing the transducer of an ventriculostomy and units of measure used to record ICP. There are also different views regarding what is considered increased intracranial pressure with some physicians are more lenient than others.[28] Nonetheless it is reasonable to state that normal (bed-rest) ICP should be less than 10 mm Hg, and ICP needs management with an upward trend or when it passes the 20 mm Hg mark. Management of ICP is best understood as changing or eliminating the factors that increase cerebral blood volume and changing or eliminating the factors that increase CSF pressure. A CT scan is necessary to demonstrate a neurosurgical lesion that may require evacuation or to consider CSF drainage. Causes of increased ICP are shown in Table 2.1.

A numeric display of ICP and its waveform is helpful in guiding therapy. This is obtained through a ventriculostomy or a parenchymal probe. The ventriculostomy might be less reliable, and an adequate waveform may not be possible. Patients who are draining bloody CSF are at risk of clotting off the catheter, which results in no waveform or in dampening of the waveform.

Most ICP management protocols include CPP management and have targets at threshold levels of ICP <20 mm Hg and CPP 50–70 mm Hg. The target ICP that requires treatment is typically set at 20 mm Hg. Most clinical studies have found that outcome is poor if ICP is not controlled. How ICP results in poor outcome is not entirely explained and can certainly not be explained by CPP alone. A consistently increased ICP of more than 20 mm Hg in patients with traumatic head injury may result in poor outcome despite consistently maintaining CPP at more than 60 mm Hg.

As alluded to earlier, the focus is on the pressure volume curve, and the relationship is nonlinear. In other words, there is usually a large change in pressure for any change in volume. The main principle is to reduce a point on the steep part of the curve to a less-steep part of the curve, making ICP much less responsive to changes in volume. If the CPP remains <60 mm Hg, the CPP can be increased to 90–100 using vasopressors or fluid resuscitation, but never without control of ICP first.

An unusual way of treating increased intracranial pressure is by managing CPP, reducing cerebral blood volume and intravascular hydrostatic pressure. This approach (the lund protocol) includes maintenance of normal colloid pressure that would reduce intracapillary hydrostatic pressure through systemic blood pressure reduction. The cerebral blood volume is reduced using thiopental, and precapillary

Table 2.1 **Causes of Increased Intracranial Pressure**

- Cerebral edema
- Mass lesion
- Acute hydrocephalus
- Cerebral vasodilation
- Cerebral venous sinus thrombosis
- Status epilepticus
- Increased intrathoracic or intraabdominal pressure
- Hyperthermia or febrile states

vasoconstriction is used to create vasoconstriction using dihydroergotamine. This protocol is not proven to be better than ICP-targeted management.[11] The protocol reduces mean arterial blood pressure to reduce intracranial volume—and thus ICP—while maintaining microcirculation with drugs such as clonidine. The Lund protocol will accept a CPP of <50 mm Hg if it will reduce ICP.

Increasing the mean arterial blood pressure may increase the CPP, but increased cerebral blood volume as a result of increased CPP can worsen edema if autoregulation is impaired. If autoregulation is intact, increased blood volume will lead to vasoconstriction, which can then result in a decrease in intracranial pressure; however, it is usually impossible to tell without sophisticated monitoring whether autoregulation is present or impaired.

Taking all protocols together, differences in neurologic outcome were not apparent when an ICP-driven management was compared with a CPP-driven management in patients with traumatic head injury. But even more surprising ICP monitoring may not be helpful if patients are aggressively treated on the basis of clinical findings (reduced consciousness) and CT abnormalities (brain edema or mass effect). Recently, ICP monitoring has been studied in traumatic brain injury in a clinical trial comparing ICP-guided management with no ICP-guided management in mostly young comatose males with severe traumatic brain injury on CT scan, nearly half of whom had upper brainstem injury. ICP monitoring and management based on ICP values did not improve outcome when compared with ICP management based on clinical judgment. ICP monitoring increased the use of barbiturates significantly.[4]

How can we best systematically approach increased ICP? The first measure is 30 degrees head elevation while avoiding any jugular venous obstruction. Next, patients should have a good oxygen saturation with SPO_2 >97% and $PaCO_2$ should be normal or low normal. This is then followed by 20% mannitol (1–2 g/kg infusion) until the plasma osmolality reaches 320 mm/L. The plasma osmolality should be closely monitored, but fortunately the risk of renal failure with mannitol—previously known as "osmotic nephrosis" and possibly due to arterial vasoconstriction—seems low in patients with normal prior renal function and no other administered potentially nephrotoxic agents.[9] Mannitol presents a major risk of inducing renal failure if the patient has intravascular volume depletion.[19] The osmolal gap (Osm calculated - Osm measured) should be measured, and mannitol should be discontinued if the gap is higher than 50 mOsmol/kg. Close monitoring for the development of hypokalemia, hyponatremia, hypocalcemia, and hypophosphatemia is needed while using high doses of mannitol.[18,30]

There is a tendency to proceed with hypertonic saline as soon as possible, which is usually limited by the presence of a central catheter. A peripherally inserted central catheter should be placed before hypertonic saline can be used. Hypertonic saline can cause significant phlebitis in high concentrations, defined as more than 3% hypertonic saline. Normally, 30 cc's of 23.4% hypertonic saline followed by repeated doses every 4 hours are used to treat increasing intracranial pressure.

The aim is to cause hypernatremia between 150 and 155 mmol/L. Continuous infusion of 1.5% hypertonic saline can be considered, although infusion of 3% hypertonic saline may cause significant fluid retention and pulmonary edema in susceptible patients. The next step is to introduce hyperventilation that reduces the $PaCO_2$ to the low 30s. Its effect is short and concerns about adverse effects (ischemia in vasoconstricted areas) with long term use have remained.

Temperature can be reduced to 34–35 Celsius using known cooling methods and antipyretic drugs. The use of therapeutic hypothermia or fever control has become a likely very effective treatment of increased intracranial pressure. Surface cooling with devices that achieve a certain target temperature is effective and may control increased intracranial pressure in patients with refractory ICP.[31] Shivering will have to be treated aggressively, because shivering can increase ICP and promote plateau waves. Shivering can be countered with buspirone 20 mg through the nasogastric tube, dexmedetomidine, IV meperidine, or IV clonidine. (The dose of dexmedetomidine is 0.4–1.5 mcg/kg per hour. The dose of meperidine is 0.4 mg/kg IV every 4 hours. The dose of clonidine is usually 3 mcg/kg in repeated doses.)

It is often forgotten that good ICP control may be achieved with adequate sedation. However, this may lead to a loss of neurologic examination; and thus there is a trade-off. Adequate sedation often can be started with intravenous propofol but typically without a bolus to avoid—expected—hypotension. Maintenance with propofol between 10 and 50 mcg/kg per minute is usually very successful in sedating the patient. Adding an analgesic agent (e.g., intravenous fentanyl) should be completely avoided. Most patients who need sedation for increasing intracranial pressure are comatose and will have less pain sensation. Intravenous opioids (e.g., fentanyl) will make a neurologic examination quite difficult. The use of IV fentanyl is only indicated if the patient is bucking the ventilator, if there is significant tachypnea, or if there is mechanical ventilator dyssynchrony. Finally, continuous EEG monitoring may be necessary to exclude the presence of ongoing seizures that could potentially increase ICP. Antiepileptic drugs may be needed.

If these interventions are unsuccessful, decompressive craniectomy should be considered. Very few clinicians are using barbiturates because of its cardiodepressant effect, significant systemic hypotension with incremental use of vasopressors or inotropes, and its very long elimination half-life that may be up to two days in certain circumstances. Nonetheless, pentobarbital can reduce intracranial pressure when a patient is loaded at 10 mg/kg IV infusion followed by maintenance of 1–3 mg/kg per hour using burst suppression as a target on EEG.

Putting It All Together

- With increasing intracranial volume, the pressure/volume curve of the intracranial contents rapidly becomes exponential
- ICP value and waveform provide useful information on brain physiology

- Continuous monitoring provides the opportunity to construct mathematical indices that can be correlated with other forms of biochemical monitoring
- Uncontrolled ICP leads to global ischemia and brainstem injury
- ICP treatment involves osmotic drugs or decompressive neurosurgery
- ICP-guided therapy may not improve outcome in traumatic brain injury

---

BY THE WAY

- Mannitol is the most commonly used first-line osmotic agent
- Hypertonic saline may have a better safety profile if used short term
- Hypertonic saline does not cause large osmotic shifts
- One large bolus of hypertonic saline may cause phlebitis
- If indicated CSF diversion using a ventriculostomy controls ICP best

---

INTRACRANIAL PRESSURE BY THE NUMBERS

- ~ 20% of patients with refractory ICP cannot be controlled eventually
- ~ 10% of intraparenchymal ICP monitors cause hemorrhage with coagulopathy
- ~ 5% of ventriculostomes cause cerebral hemorrhage
- ~ 5% of intraparenchymal ICP monitors drift after one week
- ~ 3% of intraparenchymal ICP monitors malfunction

References

1. Albeck MJ, Borgesen SE, Gjerris F, et al. Intracranial pressure and cerebrospinal fluid outflow conductance in healthy subjects. *J Neurosurg* 1991;74:597–600.
2. Avezaat CJ, van Eijndhoven JH, Wyper DJ. Cerebrospinal fluid pulse pressure and intracranial volume-pressure relationships. *J Neurol Neurosurg Psychiatry* 1979;42:687–700.
3. Budohoski KP, Czosnyka M, de Riva N, et al. The relationship between cerebral blood flow autoregulation and cerebrovascular pressure reactivity after traumatic brain injury. *Neurosurgery* 2012;71:652–660.
4. Chestnut RM, Temkin N, Carney N, et al. A trial of intracranial-pressure monitoring in traumatic brain injury. *N Engl J Med* 2012;367: 2471–2481
5. Czosnyka M, Brady K, Reinhard M, Smielewski P, Steiner LA. Monitoring of cerebrovascular autoregulation: facts, myths, and missing links. *Neurocrit Care* 2009;10:373–386.
6. Czosnyka M, Pickard JD. Monitoring and interpretation of intracranial pressure. *J Neurol Neurosurg Psychiatry* 2004;75: 813–821.
7. Czosnyka M, Richards HK, Czosnyka Z, et al. Vascular components of cerebrospinal fluid compensation. *J Neurosurg* 1999;90:752–759.
8. Czosnyka M, Smielewski P, Timofeev I, et al. Intracranial pressure: more than a number. *Neurosurg Focus* 2007;22:E10.
9. De Assis Aquino Gondim F, Aiyagari V, Shackleford A, et al. Osmolality not predictive of mannitol-induced acute renal insufficiency. *J Neurosurg* 2005;103:444–447.

10. Freshman SP, Battistella FD, Matteucci M, Wisner DH. Hypertonic saline (7.5%) versus mannitol: a comparison for treatment of acute head injuries. *J Trauma* 1993;35:344–348.
11. Grände PO. The "Lund Concept" for treatment of severe head trauma: physiological principles and clinical application. *Intensive Care Med* 2006;32:1475–1484.
12. Horn P, Münch E, Vajkoczy P, et al. Hypertonic saline solution for control of elevated intracranial pressure in patients with exhausted response to mannitol and barbiturates. *Neurol Res* 1999;21:758–764.
13. Huang SJ, Chang L, Han YY, Lee YC, Tu YK. Efficacy and safety of hypertonic saline solutions in the treatment of severe head injury. *Surg Neurol* 2006;65:539–546.
14. Juul N, Morris GF, Marshall SB, Marshall LF. Intracranial hypertension and cerebral perfusion pressure: influence on neurological deterioration and outcome in severe head injury. The Executive Committee of the International Selfotel Trial. *J Neurosurg* 2000;92:1–6.
15. Lazaridis C, Neyens R, Bodle J, DeSantis SM. High-osmolarity saline in neurocritical care: systematic review and meta-analysis. *Crit Care Med* 2013;41:1353–1360.
16. Lewis PM, Smielewski P, Rosenfeld JV, Pickard JD, Czosnyka M. Monitoring of the association between cerebral blood flow velocity and intracranial pressure. *Acta Neurochir Suppl* 2012;114:147–151.
17. Löfgren J, von Essen C, Zwetnow NN. The pressure-volume curve of the cerebrospinal fluid space in dogs. *Acta Neurol Scand* 1973;49:557–574.
18. Marko NF. Hyperosmolar therapy for intracranial hypertension: time to dispel antiquated myths. *Is J Respir Crit Care Med* 2012;185:467–468.
19. Lundberg N. Continuous recording and control of ventricular fluid pressure in neurosurgical practice. *Acta Psychiatr Scand Suppl* 1960;36:1–193.
20. Marko NF. Hypertonic saline, not mannitol, should be considered gold-standard medical therapy for intracranial hypertension. *Crit Care* 2012;16:113.
21. Marmarou A, Maset AL, Ward JD, et al. Contribution of CSF and vascular factors to elevation of ICP in severely head-injured patients. *J Neurosurg* 1987;66:883–890.
22. Menon DK. Cerebral protection in severe brain injury: physiological determinants of outcome and their optimization. *Br Med Bull* 1999;55:226–258.
23. Miller JD, Stanek A, Langfitt TW. Concepts of cerebral perfusion pressure and vascular compression during intracranial hypertension. *Prog Brain Res* 1972;35:411–432.
24. Miller JD. Volume and pressure in the craniospinal axis. *Clin Neurosurg* 1975;22:76–105.
25. Mirski AM, Denchev ID, Schnitzer SM, Hanley FD. Comparison between hypertonic saline and mannitol in the reduction of elevated intracranial pressure in a rodent model of acute cerebral injury. *J Neurosurg Anesthesiol* 2000;12:334–344.
26. Mortazavi MM, Romeo AK, Deep A, et al. Hypertonic saline for treating raised intracranial pressure: literature review with meta-analysis. *J Neurosurg* 2012;116:210–221.
27. Nakagawa K, Chang CW, Koenig MA, Yu M, Tokumaru S. Treatment of refractory intracranial hypertension with 23.4% saline in children with severe traumatic brain injury. *J Clin Anesth* 2012;24:318–323.
28. Olson DM, Batjer HH, Abdulkadir K, et al. Measuring and monitoring ICP in neurocritical care: Results from a national practice survey. *Neurocrit Care* 2014; in press.
29. Robertson CS, Valadka AB, Hannay HJ, Contant CF, Gopinath SP, Cormio M, Uzura M, Grossman RG, et al. Prevention of secondary ischemic insults after severe head injury. *Crit Care Med* 1999;27:2086–2095.
30. Ropper AH. Hyperosmolar therapy for raised intracranial pressure. *N Engl J Med* 2012;367:746–752.
31. Sadaka F, Veremakis C. Therapeutic hypothermia for the management of intracranial hypertension in severe traumatic brain injury: A systematic review. *Brain Inj* 2012;26:899–908.
32. Torre-Healy A, Marko NF, Weil RJ. Hyperosmolar therapy for intracranial hypertension. *Neurocrit Care* 2012;17:117–130.
33. Treggiari MM, Schutz N, Yanez ND, Romand JA. Role of intracranial pressure values and patterns in predicting outcome in traumatic brain injury: a systematic review. *Neurocrit Care* 2007;6:104–112.
34. Weed LH. Some limitations of the Monro–Kellie hypothesis. *Arch Surg* 1929;18:1049–1068.

3

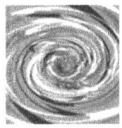

Neurology of Cerebrospinal Fluid

Cerebrospinal fluid (CSF) is found everywhere in the nervous system but primarily in the ventricles, spinal canal, and subarachnoid spaces. A major part of CSF is compartmentalized, circulates, and maintains a certain volume and pressure. Simply put, CSF circulates via a mechanism of bulk flow and is influenced by arterial pulsations, postural change, and cilia movements of the ependyma. During its circulation, it may clear the brain from metabolic byproducts. CSF volume is a result of constant CSF production (about 20 mL per hour or ½ liter daily) but is also removed at a similar rate. CSF pressure is determined by impedances at multiple locations.

Obstruction in this circulation, results in the ventricles to enlarge which may occur at any site.[18] For example, after subarachnoid hemorrhage, obstruction may occur at the basal cisterns, intraventricular foramen due to intraventricular hemorrhage, or at the level of the arachnoid granulations. In many causes of acute brain injury, acute ventricular enlargement (hydrocephalus) is an independent predictor of poor outcome. Ventricular drainage may control ICP, but it may not consistently improve level of consciousness, suggesting direct irreversible tissue damage from acute hydrocephalus. Moreover, marked dilatation of the fourth ventricle has been identified as an important indicator of poor outcome, confirming the impression that sudden massive enlargement causes damage to the periaqueductal area. Knowledge of the anatomical route of CSF flow is needed to understand mechanisms of obstruction. The changing composition of CSF in disease processes is equally important. Moreover, the CSF compartment is part of the intracranial compartment and, therefore, cannot be viewed as a separate unit without discussing the other compartments.

The clinically relevant questions to ask here are: How do we measure and interpret CSF pressure? What are clinical conditions associated with CSF hypotension and hypertension? How do we monitor and troubleshoot a ventriculostomy and lumbar drain? When is a permanent CSF drain required?

The anatomy and physiology of cerebrospinal fluid is of interest in many disease processes. In this chapter, we will discuss how to reduce increased intracranial pressure (ICP) through manipulation of spinal fluid dynamics, and discuss the changes of CSF in disease processes.

Principles

The normal pressure of CSF is 50–200 cm H_2O or 5–15 mm Hg. Approximately 5 to 7 mm Hg is just enough to overcome the pressure in the sagittal sinuses, allowing absorption. The contribution of CSF to brain physiology is at least threefold. First, despite the small volume, CSF basically allows the brain to float so that the brain's weight in effect is only a fraction of its true weight. This may minimize the effect of trauma of the brain against the skull. The brain "sags" if the CSF volume and pressure is low, and this may become clinically relevant. Second, the CSF most likely removes extra cell or waste products, mostly CO_2, lactate and hydrogen ions, and participates in immunologic transport. Third, CSF distributes biologically active substances such as the thyrotropin-releasing hormone from the hypothalamus.[5,6,7]

Harvey Cushing famously called the CSF compartment the third circulation, but it has also been considered an "intermediary between blood and nerve tissue." Cushing felt it was somewhat like blood flow and somewhat like lymphatic flow. The relationship of CSF with the venous and arterial circulation is shown in Figure 3.1. In regard to the venous circulation, it is clear that any major change in venous pressure results in CSF back-up pressure.

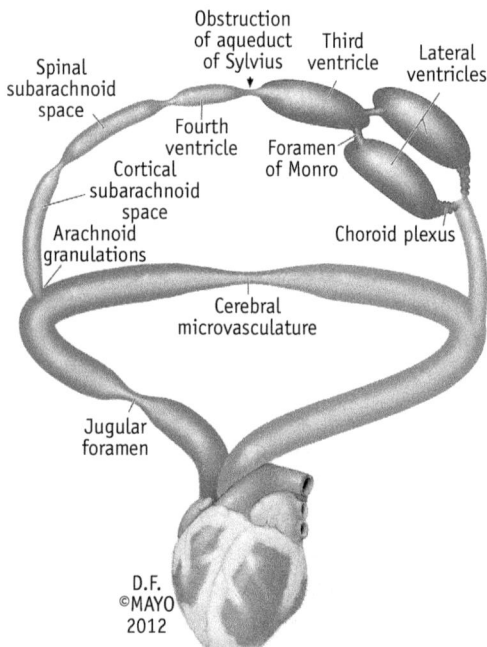

Figure 3.1 CSF in relation to venous and arterial circulation (adapted from reference 22).

There is also a resistance to CSF outflow with different maneuvers and manipulation of the cerebral vasculature. The tone of cerebral vessels influences the CSF compensatory reserve. With vasodilatation of the cerebral vasculature, compliance of the cerebrospinal compartment decreases. During hypotension resulting in decrease in the tone of all cerebral blood vessels, compliance of the arterial wall increases, resulting in increased pulse transmission from the arterial blood pressure to the ICP waveform. The resistance to CSF outflow decreases with hypotension but increases with hypercapnia. Hypercapnia may narrow the CSF flow pathway due to brain expansion (e.g., caused by an increase in cerebral blood volume).[8] The CSF relationship with arterial circulation also becomes relevant with the use of hyperosmolar therapy. The osmolality of blood and CSF is similar and approximately 295 mOsm/L. As an aside mannitol is excluded from CSF and the brain more than any other agent. The new osmotic gradient between blood and the brain, created by introducing 20% solution of mannitol, causes water to move from the extracellular space of the brain into the intravascular space.

CEREBROSPINAL FLUID BIOCHEMISTRY

The choroid plexus consists of villous folds. The choroid plexus "secretes" CSF, but basically it is a capillary network moving plasma over fenestrated epithelial cells into the ventricles using transport systems (Figure 3.2). CSF is mostly water—and certainly looks like it—but its composition is considered to be the result of different types of transport mechanisms, with a narrow regulated ion transport of sodium, chloride, bicarbonate, and calcium into the cerebrospinal fluid.[15,23] Recently discovered water channels (aquaporins) located in ependymal cells and astrocytes facilitate water transport from CSF to brain parenchyma.[21]

Sodium, as with many other compartments, is the major active cation in CSF, and there are active transport mechanisms. Although there is a balanced entry of solute and water at the choroid plexus, the calcium, magnesium, and chloride concentrations are different. Calcium in the CSF concentration is approximately half the serum level. Magnesium concentrations and chloride concentrations are higher in the CSF than in the serum. CSF has a low concentration of protein, which is much more concentrated in serum than in CSF.[15]

Glucose transport into the CSF is by facilitated diffusion, and normally CSF glucose concentrations are approximately 60% of the serum glucose value.[9] Changes of glucose in the serum are not identical to those in CSF and depend on the time measured. Changes in the serum glucose are followed by several hours of delay before the CSF glucose concentration changes. There is also an important difference in the pH in CSF and serum (the CSF pH averages 7.30 and the serum pH is 7.40).

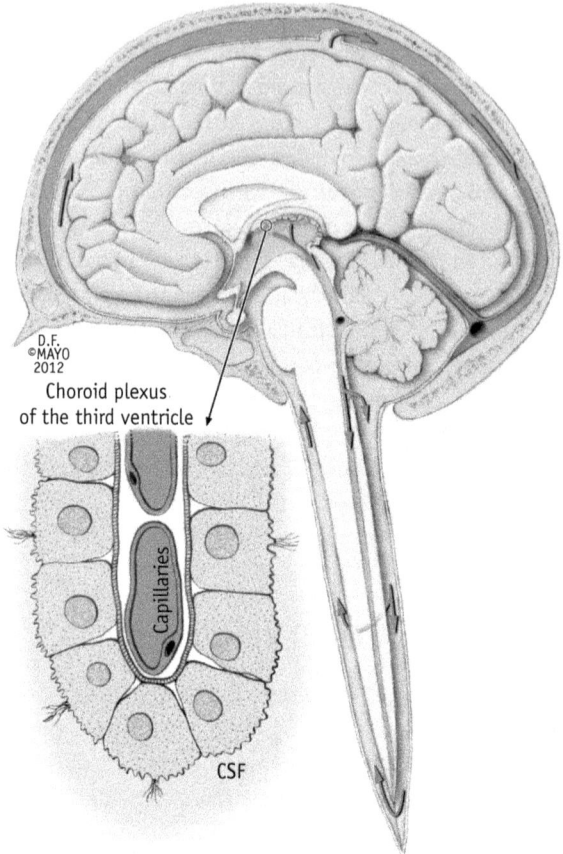

Figure 3.2 Choroid plexus showing filtration from capillaries.

CEREBROSPINAL FLUID PRESSURE RELATIONSHIPS

Intracranial pressure (ICP) depends on CSF volume and dynamics, but most of the time ICP is similar to CSF pressure.[3] As described in Chapter 2, the intracranial contents are blood, brain, and CSF and may have to accommodate another volume in pathologic circumstances. These components determine the elastance of the system (unit of pressure change per unit of volume change).

CSF has a constant production rate dependent on cerebral perfusion pressure and drains into the dural venous system using a valvular system maintaining a one-direction flow outward.[31] CSF reabsorption is dependent on CSF pressure and virtually nonexistent with CSF pressure <5 mm Hg. CSF is very position dependent; when the body is upright, venous blood in cortical veins draws into the jugular vein. As a result, CSF drains more easily into the spinal arachnoid space and may even become negative—one of the reasons valves are used in permanent ventriculoperitoneal CSF shunts.

The total volume of CSF in humans is only 100–300 mL.[27] After the CSF is formed by the choroid plexus of the lateral ventricles, it passes through the foramen of Monro into the third ventricle, which then adds more fluid by the choroid plexus in this ventricle. CSF then flows through the narrow aqueduct of Sylvius to the fourth ventricle, where a sheet-like choroid plexus adds more CSF. Fluid exits into the basal cistern and then into the subarachnoid space over the surface of the cortex. Fluid may also drain back into blood via the arachnoid granulations into the superior sagittal sinus. Systolic caudal movements of brainstem causes a wave of CSF into the spinal canal.[28] Some CSF may return via the spinal nerve roots and olfactory tracts (Figure 3.3). CSF absorption is still assumed to be at the dural venous sinuses, but lymphatic drainage into the paranasal sinuses has been considered as an additional pathway.

CSF volume can be manipulated by decreasing CSF production; this can be achieved, for example, with carbonic anhydrase inhibitors such acetazolamide.[22]

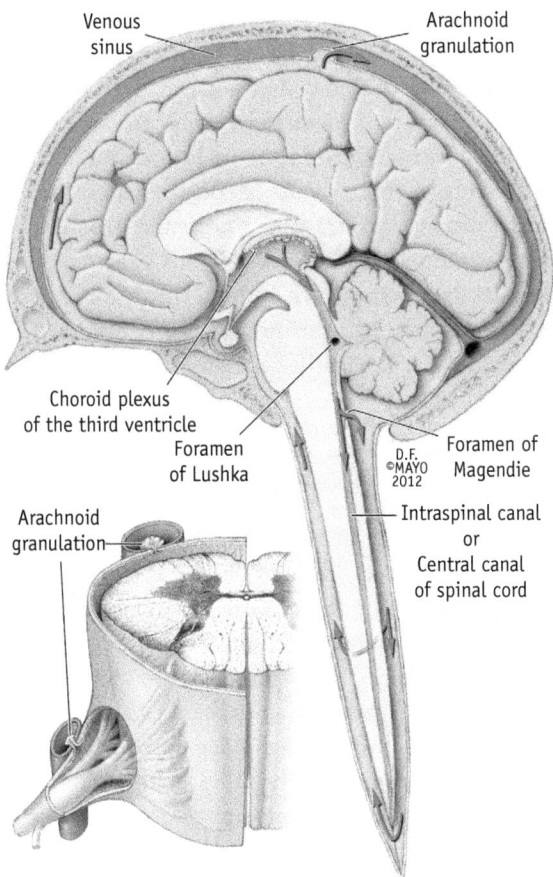

Figure 3.3 CSF circulation pathways (insert shows absorption by spinal arachnoid villi).

Improved absorption may be achieved by using corticosteroids to reduce the inflammatory response in arachnoid villi or by removing obstruction, such as a tumor.[12,13]

The CSF pressure is a function of the rate of CSF formation, the resistance to CSF absorption, and the dural sinus pressure. The contribution of dural sinus pressure in the total ICP is very large. Marmarou proposed the following equation:[18] ICP = If × R_0 + Pd (If = fluid formation, R_0 = fluid resistance, Pd = dural pressure). The changes in these components may be independent of each other. Absorption of CSF is linearly related to CSF pressure. CSF has a pulse pressure that has to overcome a certain resistance. Increased resistance to CSF outflow is a major contributor to elevated baseline ICP, and there is typically a linear relationship between resistance and ICP.[1,17]

In summary, CSF circulates from the site of secretion at the choroid plexus of the lateral ventricles toward the ventral cavities and in a rostrocaudal flow in the ventricles but in multidirectional flow in the subarachnoid spaces to the cisterna magna, through the foramen of Magendie of the fourth ventricle, and then through the craniospinal subarachnoid spaces. In the cranial subarachnoid space, it flows toward the arachnoid villi in the wall of the venous sinuses, where it is absorbed. This explains why increased venous pressure increases CSF pressure: Venous outflow obstruction leads to increased venous pressure followed by reduced CSF pressure gradient at the absorption sites, leading to decreased CSF absorption and increasing intracranial pressure. A typical scenario is cerebral venous thrombosis. CSF is also absorbed by the olfactory mucosa and cranial nerves. (These cranial nerves sheath then drain through the lymphatic system.) CSF circulating in the spinal subarachnoid space is absorbed by the epidural venous plexus and spinal nerve sheathes entering the lymphatic system.

In Practice

To determine whether there is an abnormal CSF dynamic or composition, we combine clinical findings with the results of CSF analysis (lumbar puncture or ventriculostomy) and ventricular size on CT scan into unified diagnosis. CSF circulation is abnormal in two clinical situations: (1) acute obstructive hydrocephalus,[32] and (2) acute CSF leakage. This requires acute intervention. CSF pressure manipulation may also be used in acute spinal cord ischemia.[14]

The clinical presentation of hydrocephalus depends on how quickly the obstruction evolves over time. Obstruction of the CSF results in ventricular dilation and starts proximally showing enlarging temporal horns. Acute hydrocephalus may suddenly decompensate and may be very dramatic in presentation. It is unclear why some patients with an acute hydrocephalus but alert at presentation suddenly become comatose, and triggers can rarely be identified. In some patients with fourth ventricle ependymoma, a hemorrhage in the tumor may expand the lesion and push patients over the edge. Respiratory arrest may occur from a sudden rise in ICP—as is occasionally seen in an acutely obstructed colloid cyst in the third ventricle.

Acute hydrocephalus presents invariably with a decline in consciousness and can be profound. Patients need constant prodding to open eyes, and some show purposeful motor movements only if a pain stimulus is applied. Rapidly developing stupor likely results from pressure of the expanding third ventricle on the thalami and on the ascending reticular activating system at the level of the aqueduct. With further enlargement, compression of the upper brainstem by an enlarged third ventricle occurs. Tumors that obstruct the ventricles may produce clinical signs of compression from their own mass effect. In a Parinaud syndrome the lesion is in the dorsal midbrain (pretectum) and interrupts the supranuclear mechanisms for upward gaze next to impaired convergence and a light-near dissociation of the pupillary light reflex (pupil constriction to accommodation, not to light). Pupil size changes with acute hydrocephalus, usually becoming small, likely as a result of sympathetic dysfunction at a diencephalic level. Downward gaze is not common in acute hydrocephalus in adults and is a sign of long-standing hydrocephalus.

Most patients with a rapid onset of increased CSF pressure will develop changes in breathing pattern from Cheyne-Stokes breathing to central hyperventilation. Papilledema and splinter hemorrhages may be seen, but this is a result of long-standing increased CSF pressure and therefore remains an unreliable clinical finding. CT scan shows the degree of hydrocephalus and in many instances the obstructing lesion (blood or mass). Usually, the largest parts of the ventricular system (the anterior horns of the lateral ventricles) enlarge first together with the temporal horns, and then the third and fourth ventricles—this rostrocaudal sequence was first proposed by Milhorat.[19] When hydrocephalus has developed over weeks, subependymal effusions are the best evidence of increased CSF pressure. When the fourth ventricle is normal, the obstruction is at the third ventricle level and can be from a suprasellar tumor not readily identified on CT. Magnetic resonance imaging is urgently needed to explain the obstruction.

It is not readily appreciated that acute hydrocephalus on CT may not always explain all clinical findings. Coma in aneurysmal subarachnoid hemorrhage with acute hydrocephalus may be caused by diffuse global ischemic injury from massively increased intracranial pressure and markedly reduced cerebral perfusion pressure, and not all patients improve rapidly with a ventriculostomy placement. CSF obstruction leads to increased intracranial pressure, which in turn reduces cerebral perfusion pressure. When CSF/ICP increases to a certain threshold—mostly in the range of 40 mm Hg—cerebral perfusion pressure closes down and global ischemia occurs. Massive hemorrhage into the thalamus may be associated with large hemoventricle casts, but patients will not awaken after CSF diversion because the thalamocortical connections are destroyed.

The intervention in acute hydrocephalus obviously is to rapidly reduce CSF volume and pressure (Figure 3.4). CSF can be diverted with an external catheter or internal catheter (ventriculoperitoneal shunt). CSF diversion usually involves placement of a ventriculostomy, and CSF escapes at certain threshold ICP levels. The ventricular catheters are connected to a transducer that allows continuous ICP readings. The system is a closed system and all connections should be tightened to maintain integrity. The main system stopcock is placed at the tragus of the ear (assumed to be foramen of Monro). The handle of the stopcock determines flow. When the handle is turned in the direction of the port, that port is closed. (To open, turn handle to operator; to close, turn to patient. Another way to remember is open drainage system nine o'clock position; closed at three o'clock position.) A 12-hour position will drain and monitor, but should be avoided. CSF can be inspected, and opening up the stopcock will show pulsating CSF—closing will result in transducing CSF pressure, and waveform (Chapter 2) will become apparent. One side port is used for continuous drainage and sampling. The drip chamber can be moved up and down and placed at a desired level against the zero-reference-level stopcock. The drip chamber at the end of the drain line is typically fixed by a 15-cm length of pressure tubing

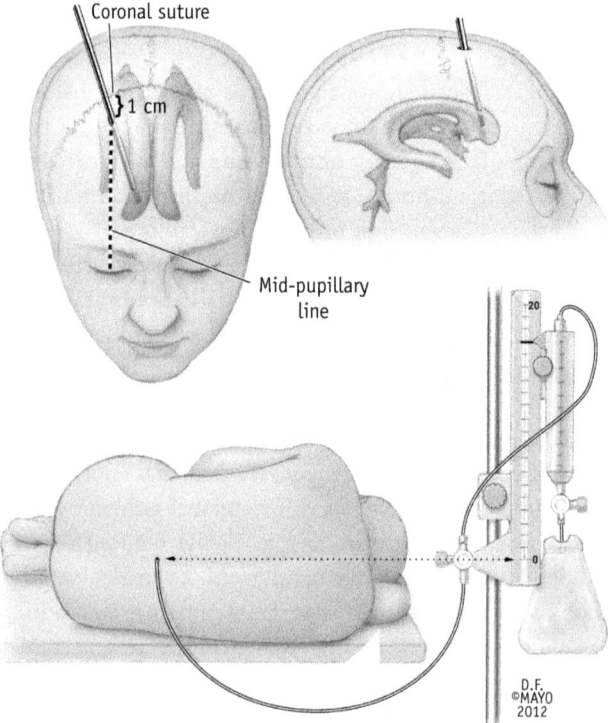

Figure 3.4 CSF diversion techniques (ventricular and lumbar).

to secure drainage in the drip chamber when the ICP rises above 15 mm Hg. Abnormal resorption of cerebrospinal fluid can be assumed when the daily yield of cerebrospinal fluid approximates 200 mL with a drip chamber at a level of 20 cm H_2O. All ports are closed before movement of the patient, including turning or transfer to a cart.

An intraventricular catheter based on a fluid-filled system has the major disadvantage of dampening the system, which makes readings less reliable. This may become a problem when progressive cerebral edema collapses the ventricles, positioning the catheter against the ventricular wall.

The ventricular drainage system may have no drainage, and further lowering the drainage system below the foramen of Monro may have no effect. Commonly, the system becomes blocked when fully filled (casting) with blood. An occluded catheter can be irrigated with small amounts of sterile isotonic saline. Frequently, however, dampening of the waveform suggests an air bubble. Air bubbles in the system can be eliminated by withdrawing air from the monitoring line, but only after the system to the patient is closed. Irrigation of the drain may be needed to remove brain tissue (as a result of prior very high ICP pressure) or blood clots (cerebral hemorrhage with massive intraventricular filling). The troubleshooting procedure is first to flush the tubing (away from the patient) and then, if unsuccessful, to change the entire drainage system. This also has to be done if there has been a disconnection, which significantly increases the chance of infection. Flushing is best performed with 0.5–2 mL of isotonic sodium chloride. Thrombolytics are possibly helpful (2 ml of 1 mg/ml tPA mixture) and several doses (12-hour interval) may be needed to sort effect. It has a good safety profile even in a higher dose of 3 mg every 12 hours.[20]

Using antibiotics may reduce infection risk. The risk of ventriculitis is variable but highest in patients with intraventricular hemorrhage, ICP higher than 20 mm Hg, placement longer than 5 days, frequent CSF sampling or manipulation, and disconnection of the system. Irrigation with thrombolytics also increases the risk. There is some benefit to using prophylactic antibiotics, but there may be a risk with prolonged use of broad-spectrum antibiotics.[27]

Hemorrhagic complications with ventriculostomy are variable in the published literature.[2] Use of subcutaneous low-molecular-weight heparin and warfarin increases the risk, but the number of clinically significant hemorrhages remains estimated around 1%, doubling with full anticoagulation. It is not known whether reduction of this risk may be potentially offset by increased deep venous thrombosis and pulmonary embolism.

Acute hydrocephalus may also be managed with placement of a lumbar drain (Figure 3.4). There are contraindications, and any hemispheric or extracranial hematoma with mass effect or shift of midline structures may worsen with acute reduction of CSF volume (most reduction may be during placement). A lumbar drain is also a concern in patients with an obstructive clot in the third or fourth ventricle. As in a ventriculostomy, a coagulopathy (INR > 1.4 or PTT > 1.5 times control or platelets less than 70,000) should be excluded. Placement is simple through a lumbar puncture needle but may require fluoroscopy. The collection chamber of a lumbar drain is placed at the level of the shoulder (and not at the tragus, as is often erroneously done), and typically 10–20 cc of CSF is drained per hour.

Increased CSF volume can also be reduced by acetazolamide,[22] furosemide, and corticosteroids. Acetazolamide inhibits carbonic anhydrase–mediated CSF production and this can be quite substantial, up to 50% of normal production. Nonetheless, the effect of acetazolamide is of short duration and not clinically useful in the long run. The decision to remove the ventriculostomy is determined by whether a normal ICP can be achieved, whether there are small volumes of CSF drainage at certain levels, and whether there is no change in ventricle size with raising the level of the drain, but most importantly lack of clinical deterioration with clamping of the brain. A permanent ventriculoperitoneal shunt will have to be placed if the above criteria are not fulfilled. Depending on the site of the obstruction (aqueduct of Sylvius, foramen, ventricle), a third ventriculotomy can be performed. Clinical examples are patients with tectal tumors or congenital or acquired aqueductal stenosis. The neurosurgeon will place the endoscope into the ventricle and passes it through the lateral ventricle and foramen of Monro into the third ventricle, perforating the floor of the third ventricle (using puncture and balloon inflation). If elevation of intracranial pressure is caused by increased cerebral venous pressure, some have considered stenting of the transverse sinus if a stenosis is found.

A permanent drain contains a shunt valve that maintains an instant flow of CSF. Flow control valves with low settings may cause overdrainage and subdural effusions or hematomas, in particular if it lowers CSF below the physiologic limits (less than 5 cm H_2O). Valve settings can be programmed (from 3 to 20 cm H_2O pressures.) After permanent shunt is placed a series of X rays will document patency (it may also be needed in later presumed shunt failure to show disconnection (Figure 3.5).

A second equally important clinical problem is management of CSF hypotension, best described as spontaneous intracranial hypotension. Opening CSF pressure can be normal, decreased, or unmeasurable. This is caused by a CSF leak that can be spontaneous. A CSF leak can be a consequence of a prior craniectomy, post-traumatic CSF otorrhea or rhinorrhea.

Acute CSF leakage will result in low pressure and volume and (as mentioned before) sagging of the brain, and can be recognized by the presence of bilateral subdural hematomas on CT scan as the result of tearing of the bridging dural veins. Magnetic resonance imaging in patients with intracranial hypotension often show diffuse enhancement of the pachymeninges with gadolinium in combination with small bilateral, subdural fluid collections, a general downward displacement, bucking of the entire brain and tonsillar herniation ("cork in the

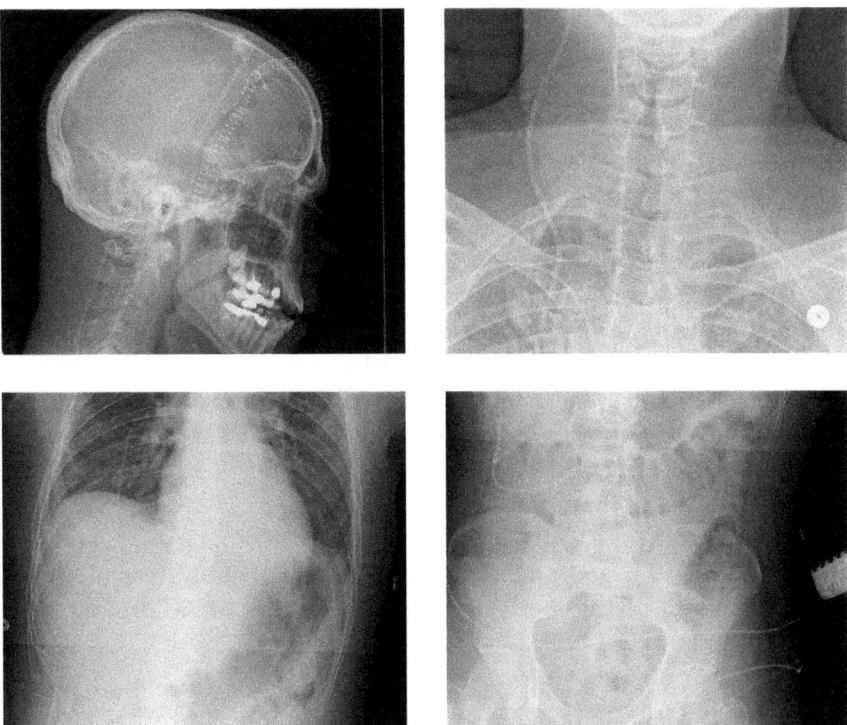

Figure 3.5 Shunt series to prove continuity of ventriculoperitoneal drain.

bottle"). CSF leaks are usually at the cervicothoracic junction or in the thoracic spine.[10,24] Bilateral posterior circulation infarcts may occur due to downward displacement of these arteries or due to compression at the tentorial edge from draping of softer brain tissue.[10] Infarcts in the pons due to basilar artery stretch has been reported.[25,26]

It has been convincingly pointed out that the concept of Monro-Kellie can be applied both with intracranial hypertension and with intracranial hypotension. With a decrease in volume of CSF, the cerebral volume will decrease and will be compensated for by increased intracranial blood volume and, thus, hyperemia, engorgement of the venous sinuses, and the well-known hyperemia of the pituitary gland although perfusion of these structures is largely provided by extracranial circulation. Meningeal hyperemia is the reason for contrast enhancement of the meninges on MRI, and similar changes are seen in the spinal canal.[19]

Clinical manifestations of spontaneous intracranial hypotension can be very serious and acute. Several reports have documented coma sometimes after several weeks of orthostatic headache (headache much worse with standing and much better with lying flat often within minutes of position change). Bilateral subdural hematomas are usually found, but surgery to evacuate them may worsen the downward displacement, reaccumulation of subdural blood, and leading to reexploration if the true mechanism is not recognized.[10,25] Management in these patients is immediate placement into a flat or Trendelenburg position. CT myelogram remains the most valuable diagnostic test. Surgical repair of the CSF leak is generally successful.[24,25]

Finally, an important therapeutic intervention should be mentioned here. CSF pressure may play a role in acute ischemic spinal cord injury in patients who underwent repair of a thoracoabdominal aneurysm.[4] If the CSF pressure in the spinal cord can be kept low, the spinal perfusion can improve. Although this practice is usually in patients at the time of thoracoabdominal aortic aneurysm surgery, the delayed onset of acute paraplegia following these types of surgeries or sudden appearance in patients with acute aortic dissection warrants consideration of CSF diversion therapy. Removal of the CSF decreases CSF pressure (which is often elevated) and improves spinal cord perfusion pressure. The best treatment is a large 40-mL CSF tap followed by a lumbar drain placement and drainage. Any patient in whom the CSF potentially can be increased might benefit from this intervention.

PUTTING IT ALL TOGETHER

- CSF moves through bulk flow and refreshes four times a day
- CSF components are all in communication
- CSF circulation has a great impact on intracranial content and compliance
- CSF dynamics are related to CSF outflow and related to dural venous pressure
- CSF diversion is the best treatment to reduce ICP
- CSF hypotension may have major clinical consequences

BY THE WAY

- Ventriculostomy and lumbar drain precludes use of full anticoagulation
- Avoid S.C. heparin for at least 24 hours after a traumatic lumbar drain placement
- Keep a lumbar drain for less than 72 hours
- Keep ventriculostomy less than 1–2 weeks
- Ventriculostomy placement and removal requires platelets $> 100 \times 10^3/\mu L^3$ and INR < 1.5.

> **CEREBROSPINAL FLUID BY THE NUMBERS**
> - ~80% of CSF is in the subarachnoid space
> - ~70% of CSF is produced in choroid plexus
> - ~60% of CSF glucose when compared to plasma
> - ~10% of total brain volume is CSF
> - ~5% of actual brain weight due to CSF presence

References

1. Albeck MJ, Børgesen SE, Gjerris F, et al. Intracranial pressure and cerebrospinal fluid outflow conductance in healthy subjects. *J Neurosurg* 1991;74:597–600.
2. Binz DD, Toussaint LG 3rd, Friedman JA. Hemorrhagic complications of ventriculostomy placement: a meta-analysis. *Neurocrit Care* 2009;10:253–256.
3. Bulat M, Klarica M. Recent insights into a new hydrodynamics of the cerebrospinal fluid. *Brain Res Rev* 2011;65:99–112.
4. Cinà CS, Abouzahr L, Arena GO, et al. Cerebrospinal fluid drainage to prevent paraplegia during thoracic and thoracoabdominal aortic aneurysm surgery: a systematic review and meta-analysis. *J Vasc Surg* 2004;40:36–44.
5. Cutler RW, Page L, Galicich J, Watters GV. Formation and absorption of cerebrospinal fluid in man. *Brain* 1968;91:707–720.
6. Cutler RW, Spertell RB. Cerebrospinal fluid: a selective review. *Ann Neurol* 1982;11:1–10.
7. Czosnyka M, Czosnyka Z, Momjian S, Pickard JD. Cerebrospinal fluid dynamics. *Physiol Meas* 2004;25:R51–76.
8. Czosnyka M, Richards HK, Czosnyka Z, et al. Vascular components of cerebrospinal fluid compensation. *J Neurosurg* 1999;90:752–759.
9. Davson H, Welch K, Segal MB. *Physiology and Pathophysiology of the Cerebrospinal Fluid.* Edinburgh, Churchill Livingstone, 1987.
10. Dhillon AK, Rabinstein AA, Wijdicks EF. Coma from worsening spontaneous intracranial hypotension after subdural hematoma evacuation. *Neurocrit Care* 2010;12:390–394.
11. Eklund A, Smielewski P, Chambers I, et al. Assessment of cerebrospinal fluid outflow resistance. *Med Biol Eng Comput* 2007;45:719–735.
12. Ekstedt J. CSF hydrodynamic studies in man. 1. Method of constant pressure CSF infusion. *J Neurol Neurosurg Psychiatry* 1977;40:105–119.
13. Ekstedt J. CSF hydrodynamic studies in man. 2. Normal hydrodynamic variables related to CSF pressure and flow. *J Neurol Neurosurg Psychiatry* 1978;41:345–353.
14. Fedorow CA, Moon MC, Mutch WA, Grocott HP. Lumbar cerebrospinal fluid drainage for thoracoabdominal aortic surgery: rationale and practical considerations for management. *Anesth Analg* 2010;111:46–58.
15. Fishman RA. *Cerebrospinal Fluid in Diseases of the Nervous System.* Philadelphia, WB Saunders Company, 1980.
16. Löfgren J. Effects of variations in arterial pressure and arterial carbon dioxide tension on the cerebrospinal fluid pressure-volume relationships. *Acta Neurol Scand* 1973;49:586–598.
17. Marmarou A, Shulman K, Rosende RM. A nonlinear analysis of the cerebrospinal fluid system and intracranial pressure dynamics. *J Neurosurg* 1978;48:332–344.
18. Milhorat TH. Acute hydrocephalus. *N Engl J Med.* 1970; 283:857–859.
19. Mokri B. The Monro-Kellie hypothesis: applications in CSF volume depletion. *Neurology* 2001;56:1746–1748.

20. Naff N, Williams MA, Keyl PM et al. Low-dose recombinant tissue-type plasminogen activator enhances clot resolution in brain hemorrhage: the intraventricular hemorrhage thrombolysis trial. *Stroke* 2011;42:3009–3016.
21. Papadopoulos MC, Verkman AS. Aquaporin water channels in the nervous system. *Nat Rev Neurosci*. 2013;14:265–277.
22. Rubin RC, Henderson ES, Ommaya AK, Walker MD, Rall DP. The production of cerebrospinal fluid in man and its modification by acetazolamide. *J Neurosurg* 1966;25:430–436.
23. Sakka L, Coll G, Chazal J. Anatomy and physiology of cerebrospinal fluid. *Eur Ann Otorhinolaryngol Head Neck Dis* 2011;128:309–316.
24. Schievink WI, Schwartz MS, Maya MM, Moser FG, Rozen TD. Lack of causal association between spontaneous intracranial hypotension and cranial cerebrospinal fluid leaks. *J Neurosurg* 2012;116:749–754.
25. Schievink WI. Spontaneous spinal cerebrospinal fluid leaks and intracranial hypotension. *JAMA* 2006;295:2286–2296.
26. Schievink WI. Stroke and death due to spontaneous intracranial hypotension. *Neurocrit Care* 2013;18:248–251.
27. Sonabend AM, Korenfeld Y, Crisman C, et al. Prevention of ventriculostomy-related infections with prophylactic antibiotics and antibiotic-coated external ventricular drains: a systematic review. *Neurosurgery* 2011;68:996–1005.
28. Srinivasan VM, O'Neill BR, Jho D, Whiting DM, Oh MY. The history of external ventricular drainage. *J Neurosurg* 2014, in press.
29. Symss NP, Oi S. Theories of cerebrospinal fluid dynamics and hydrocephalus: historical trend. *J Neurosurg Pediatrics* 2013;11:170–177.
30. Sullivan HG, Allison JD. Physiology of cerebrospinal fluid. In: Wilkins RH, Rengahary SS, eds. *Neurosurgery*. New York, McGraw-Hill, 1985. Vol. 3, 2125–2135.
31. Weiss MH, Wertman N. Modulation of CSF production by alterations in cerebral perfusion pressure. *Arch Neurol* 1978;35:527–529.
32. Welch K. The principles of physiology of the cerebrospinal fluid in relation to hydrocephalus including normal pressure hydrocephalus. *Adv Neurol* 1975;13:247–332.

4

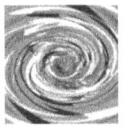

Neurology of Unconsciousness

When we are conscious we are awake, alert, vigilant, aware, having thoughts and intentions. When we become unconscious we expect a nothingness. Explaining consciousness is a supreme complex problem and there is no a unified model. Neuroscientists and physicians like to interpret consciousness as an anatomical and neurophysiologic system involving conceptual modules from attributes such as the limbic system (emotion and motivation), the temporal lobes and hippocampal systems (memory), the prefrontal cortex (execution), and other association cortices (processing).[58] These neuronal circuits and networks operate using neurotransmitters. In all of it there is a preeminence of the brainstem.[23,38,39]

Disorders of consciousness can be expected when acute brain injury is widespread. After any major neurocatastrophe, patients remain afflicted by a marked disability and the level of consciousness was often used to further classify patients. Severe neurologic injury was typically dichotomized as "severe disability or persistent vegetative state." However, rehabilitation physicians recognized that patients in a supposedly persistent vegetative state (PVS) were sometimes awake at times, albeit minimally so. The patient's behavior could in fact be purposeful, but these responses could be excruciatingly slow and often inconsistent. Therefore an attempt was made to further define this condition (minimally conscious state, or MCS) and set it apart from PVS.[19,20]

There was a status quo of knowledge in disorders of consciousness until fairly recently. The emerging use of functional magnetic resonance imaging (fMRI) in these patients has been nothing short of an eye opener. Suddenly—for the world to see—hot red "functioning" areas were imaged in patients presumably diagnosed with PVS or MCI.[7,16,29]

Moreover, fMRI visualized—for the first time—brain activation with certain tasks in these patients.[14,36] Families of patients may now start to believe that with the current technological level of fMRI we can potentially find a way to communicate using a computer interface. With a major surge in modern neuroimaging, this now may become the dominating question; is there anybody in there and can we communicate goals of care?[41,57]

Any physician involved with patients with severely impaired consciousness knows too well that during this period there is very little retention of experiences, nor is there much recollection of specific events, tests or even painful moments. It is against this background information—severe brain injury leads to inability to retain impressions—that patients who survive such an ordeal should be seen. How much does a severely injured, minimally conscious patient observe and feel? How much does a patient with a clinical diagnosis of a PVS—and activation of cortices after a stimulus—observe and feel? Without a response, we will not know and may correctly or incorrectly assume—based on the severity of injury—that there is none. And vice versa with a response we could assume there truly is one. What do the results of fMRI mean, and what is going to be its role in clinical diagnosis and decision making? Are patients in a PVS, unconscious or—far more provocatively—are they unresponsive or, "functionally locked in"?[15,29,44]

This chapter provides core knowledge needed for any physician involved with the care of these patients. Better understanding of the different categories of prolonged disorders of consciousness may lead to more specific management for some patients. At this time, however, there are many unanswered questions. For now, we speak of minimally conscious state (MCS) and persistent vegetative state (PVS) and believe we know how to recognize these conditions. When examining a patient with an altered consciousness, we need to decide not only where the abnormality is located, but also how much and why—in other words, what is damaged, is this altered conscious state reversible or permanent, and what causes it.

Principles

The focus here is on describing the current understanding of the neurology of consciousness, but for practical ends. The first step is to look at the anatomical structures. The second step is to look at lesions that lead to unconsciousness.

THE NEUROANATOMY OF CONSCIOUSNESS

For the time being, awareness of the surroundings—the Cartesian *cogito ergo sum*—can possibly be explained by the contribution of several anatomical structures. A functional cortex is a sine qua non. Next to cortical activation, the four involved (and interconnected) structures are the thalamus, forebrain, posterior hypothalamus, and brainstem nuclei in the reticular formation sending fibers upward. Their function varies and there are generators, gatekeepers or filters, and on and off switches.

The most important generator is in the brainstem. The discovery of a specialized alerting system coincided with the demonstration of abnormalities in the midbrain and hypothalamus of patients with epidemic encephalitis who before they died were stuporous. This led to further studies in animals, and brainstem transection experiments could induce sleep-like states. Electrical stimulation in a drowsy animal could wake the animal. An interlacing network of fiber bundles was found in the brainstem—named the reticular alerting system—that would activate the cortex and increase muscle tone.[9,57] This structure had the main function of awaking us and alerting us to incoming information, and these neurons would then send signals to different brain structures.[26,32,35] The anatomical boundaries of the brainstem tegmentum in which specific nuclei could be involved in the maintenance of consciousness in humans have been revisited recently. The maximal area involved in coma was in the upper pontine tegmentum.[38]

The ascending activating reticular system (ARAS)—as it is now known—is stimulated by spinal and cranial nerves carrying proprioceptive, visual, and auditory information. These interconnecting cells, located in the dorsal part of the lower pons, "ascend up" with some individual bundles to the thalamus and become active during the awake state and also during rapid eye movement (REM) in sleep, playing a major role in the sleep–wake cycle.[43,51]

Another important structure is the anterior cingulate cortex. Its key role is the orchestration of attention and motivation. It functions when the persons have to make a judgment call but also have to decide with precision. Lack of initiative, economy of movement, and mutism result from its dysfunction, in which case awareness is markedly impaired.

Starting from the ARAS, two anatomical pathways have been located. One pathway projects to the thalamus and connects to the cortex via multiple loops and circuits. The other pathway synapses and ends in the posterior part of the hypothalamus, subthalamus, and basal forebrain connecting to the cortex but bypassing the thalamus (Figure 4.1).

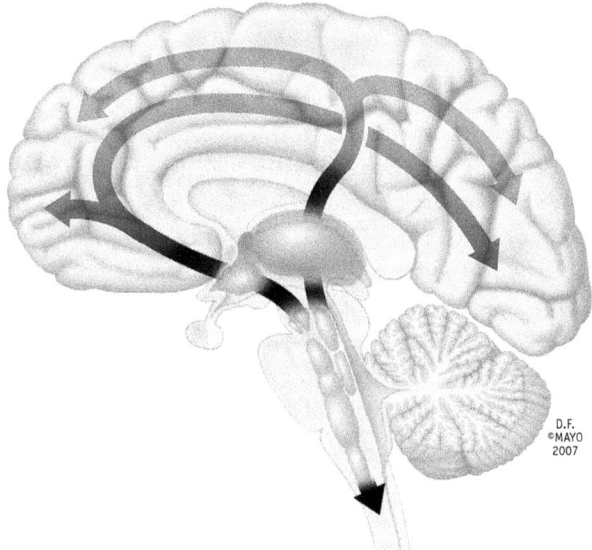

Figure 4.1 Pathways in maintaining consciousness.

The nuclei within the thalamus sort out—filter, so to speak—input from the reticular formation and limbic system structures before spreading out throughout the cortex. The thalamic reticular nucleus participates in corticothalamocortical interactions. This thalamic reticular nucleus is thus important in "gating" signals and control of the activity of other thalamic nuclei.[52]

THE NEUROCHEMISTRY OF CONSCIOUSNESS

Neurotransmitters are needed to fire up these projected neurons and to regulate wakefulness; they are located in several monoaminergic neuronal cell groups. The main neurotransmitters are norepinephrine, dopamine, serotonin, acetylcholine, histamine, and orexin-hypocretin.[49]

All the pathways project diffusely to the cortex, some with more specific targets. Norepinephrine and serotonin are very active during awake states. The substantia nigra and ventral tegmental area and retrorubral field all contain dopaminergic neurons. They ascend from the brainstem and target the forebrain, and relay in the striatum and cerebral cortex. Dopamine release is expected during aroused waking situations, and depletion of catecholamines results in hypersomnia, slowness in responsiveness, or no response at all. Dopaminergic neurons may have a more specific role in maintaining wakefulness, hence use of dopaminergic drugs (amantadine) as a treatment option.[26]

The reticular formation is largely active through the neurotransmitter glutamate. In addition, the reticular formation contains neurons that use gamma-aminobutyric acid (GABA), which has control through inhibition. The drug zolpidem potentiates the GABA receptors and would facilitate sedation, but a paradoxical effect in MCS exists in some patients for whom it is a stimulating agent.

The noradrenergic neurons are located in the locus coeruleus, with primary projection sites throughout the entire cortex, but also relaying input to the thalamus, hypothalamus, and basal forebrain. It may play a role in attention focusing. There is evidence that the noradrenergic locus coeruleus neuron mostly discharges in situations with high arousal, including stress.

The serotonergic raphe neurons use serotonin and they ascend from the midbrain raphe nucleus to the forebrain and cortex. Depletion of serotonin leads to insomnia and also an aroused waking state with increased eating and sexual behavior.

Of considerable interest are the histaminergic neurons using histamine as a neurotransmitter located in the ventral lateral posterior hypothalamus (tuberomammillary nucleus), lateral to the mamillary nuclei. The fact that antihistamines cause drowsiness indicates that histamine has an important role in waking. Histaminergic cells are also involved in cortical activation of waking. The histaminergic neurons have been found to send widespread ascending and descending tracts through areas of the brain that are known to control sleep–wake states.

The posterior hypothalamus has a plethora of neurotransmitters or neuroactive substances that include GABAergic and glutaminergic neurons, dopaminergic neurons, the neuropeptide orexin-hypocretin, and histaminergic cell bodies in the tuberomammillary nucleus. The posterior hypothalamus receives descending tracts from the preoptic anterior hypothalamus and forebrain and ascending input from the brainstem. The posterior hypothalamus has also been called the "waking center," acting mostly as an on/off switch. The site that has been identified is the preoptic area of the hypothalamus. The posterior hypothalamus, when stimulated, creates not only cortical activation but also arousal responses that include pupillary dilatation, increased respiratory rate, increased heart rate, and increased blood pressure.

There is an abundance of connectivity and only a fraction of it is understood. It remains thus important to recognize that lesions in the thalamocortical activating system or in the hypothalamic arousal system do not always produce long-standing difficulties with wakefulness. A recent study found that destruction of the thalamic neurons did not result in loss of cortical activation. Similarly, destruction of the neurons in the posterior hypothalamus did not result in waking difficulties.

THE PATHOLOGY OF UNCONSCIOUSNESS

Persistent coma is associated with widespread brain injury. Destructive lesions involving the cortex, thalamus or connecting fibers in the white matter are the major mechanisms of coma.[1] The thalamus and ARAS can also be damaged from shift and compression of these structures. The impact of lesions to these structures is substantial, leaving patients in a permanent state of unconsciousness. More selective lesions or those involving only unilateral lesions of the thalamus and upper brainstem will not impair consciousness or will affect consciousness only transiently. Involvement of the thalamus alone may lead to fluctuation of consciousness, but persistent coma is usually seen if the lesion—whether compressive or directly destructive—extends into the mesencephalon. Thalamic predominance has been reported in autopsy studies (most notorious the condition of Karen Ann Quinlan who was in PVS case). Involvement of the anterior cingulate gyrus is seldom seen in isolation, just as with lesions in the association cortex involving the precuneus and cuneus. Akinetic mutism—a condition marked by eye-open coma (or extreme unattentiveness) with eyes still intermittently fixating on objects—is the most common clinical correlate of lesions of the anterior cingulate cortex. In prolonged coma there often is secondary injury of the brainstem due to shift, torsion, compaction, and secondary vascular lesions from damage to the penetrating arteries. Sudden enlargement of the aqueduct in obstructive hydrocephalus may be another mechanism of localized brainstem injury.

When autopsy cases of patients with PVS and MCS or other severely disabled cases are compared with each other, more severe injury is found in PVS.[1] For example, in traumatic brain injury there are frequent lesions in the thalamus as well as multiple other areas of axonal injury (e.g., corpus callosum, rostral brainstem).

Anoxic-ischemic injury causing PVS usually affects the entire cortical mantle, not only all territories (with predilection for the parieto-occipital region compared with the frontotemporal region) but also throughout the full thickness, replacing neurons and nerve fibers with gliosis, lipid phagocytes, and collagen. Cavities in caudate and lentiform nucleus are common. The thalamus is also commonly involved. Purkinje cells and granular layers in the cerebellum are more commonly destroyed after anoxic-ischemic injury, and cystic softening in periaqueductal gray and dorsolateral brainstem are other pathologic findings.

TESTING UNCONSCIOUSNESS

As noted before we can expect that any change in level of arousal correlates with abnormality in the midbrain, pons, thalamus, or cortex,[48] but there is particular interest in the anterior cingulate cortex, precuneus, and cuneus. Transitions from a minimally conscious state may be related to functional improvement in these cortical locations.

Neuroimaging studies have contributed to our further understanding of wakefulness. Proton emission tomography (PET) has been used to indirectly study neuronal activity of the brain.[3,33,40,60] In these studies, cerebral blood flow is used as an indicator of neuronal activity. It assumes that increased neuronal activity induces an increase in metabolism, which then prompts a vasodilatory hemodynamic response. In addition, there is a link between the metabolic rate for oxygen and regional cerebral blood flow. PET scanning also revealed that these changes are not accompanied by changes in oxygen consumption, which increased the interest in using fMRI scan because MRI signals are sensitive to oxygenation of blood. Using fMRI, it has been proposed that the posterior cingulate, retrosplenial, and all associative cortices are important in processing of cortical information.[42,47,54] The connections observed involve not only the ARAS but also the mesiofrontal cortex, thalamus, cuneus, and precuneus.[8] This led to the concept of a "disconnection syndrome" in unconsciousness and was supported by reduced glucose metabolism as measured by PET and, contrarily, increase with improvement of consciousness.

Functional MRI of the brain is able to demonstrate engaged networks after the patient is asked to perform a task. Functional MRI is a hemodynamic modality, meaning that tissue perfusion, blood volume, and oxygen concentration change when neurons become active. It is very conceivable that signal changes on MRI are a good representation of neuronal activation; however, fMRI does not measure neuronal activity, and the blood oxygen level dependent (BOLD) signal is only a surrogate of neuronal activity. Neuronal activity converts oxyhemoglobin into deoxyhemoglobin and is followed by a compensatory increase in cerebral perfusion and this is measured as increased signal intensity.[30,31] Functional

MRI visualizes response to a sensory stimulus and it may show activation of the primary cortex in vegetative state or MCS and in disabled neurologic patients without decrease in alertness. In MCS, a much more vigorous stimulus is needed to produce activation. When vegetative state is compared with MCS, the resting state (also known as the default mode network) on fMRI in MCS shows greater connectivity and white matter integrity.

Let's look at this in more detail. This "default" network is an active system that is present only when individuals are not focused on the external environment. It was discovered when researchers measured activity in humans who had no directed mental state. It was known that the global rate of metabolism in the resting state was as active as when individuals were asked to solve complex mathematical problems. Other studies have suggested that autobiographical memory, remembering the past, and thinking about future events are all activated in this network. These networks thus could represent task-unrelated images and thoughts, or perhaps operation of self-awareness. The system, therefore, is active in passive settings and during tasks that direct attention away from external stimuli (mind-wandering). The network is deactivated with a target-directed and attention-focused processing. Most experts agree that the three-part response of the perception-thinking-action model is an oversimplification, but the BOLD signal is stronger with attention (shown in the primary visual cortex with different perceptual states).

This default mode (Figure 4.2) network includes the precuneus, temporoparietal junction, and medial prefrontal cortex, which shows "idling" activity when at

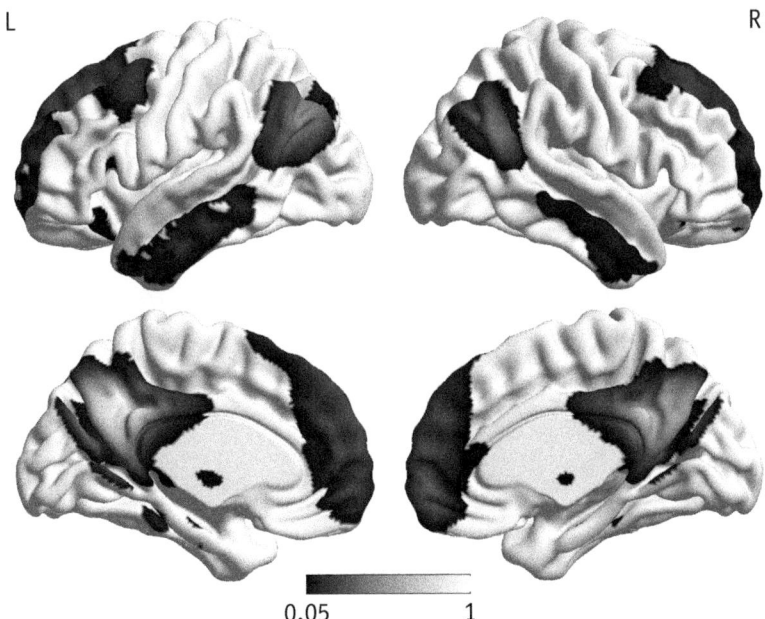

Figure 4.2 Default mode network.

rest and deactivation in task. Reduction in the functional connectivity of these brain regions has been seen in patients with altered consciousness. It is understood that absent corticothalamic connectivity has more implications than preserved corticocortical connectivity, such as that which can be seen in a patient in PVS. Others have found that the posterior portion of the default mode network is a defined characteristic of minimally conscious patients.[12,13,34] It also has become clear that abnormal functional connectivity between corticocortical and thalamocortical regions correlates with structural injury to white matter fascicles when shown with diffusion tensor imaging or tractography.[17]

The fMRI connectivity to cuneus and precuneus posterior is also much different in minimally conscious patients as compared with patients in a PVS. (In comparison, there is intact metabolism or connectivity in both the anterior posterior portion of the default mode network in patients who are classically locked-in and often have no disorder of consciousness). Some studies have shown that task-induced deactivation of the default mode network is reduced in patients with a PVS, and may improve when recovery is seen later.[37,53] Others have claimed that presence of a default mode network could indicate that coma may be reversible.[37,53] Nevertheless, the reality is that many patients in PVS will only show activation of Heschl's gyrus, without any other activation (Figure 4.3).

Patients with disorders of consciousness have been tested using different tasks, mostly responses to name calling. One group perfected "mental imaginary" tests,

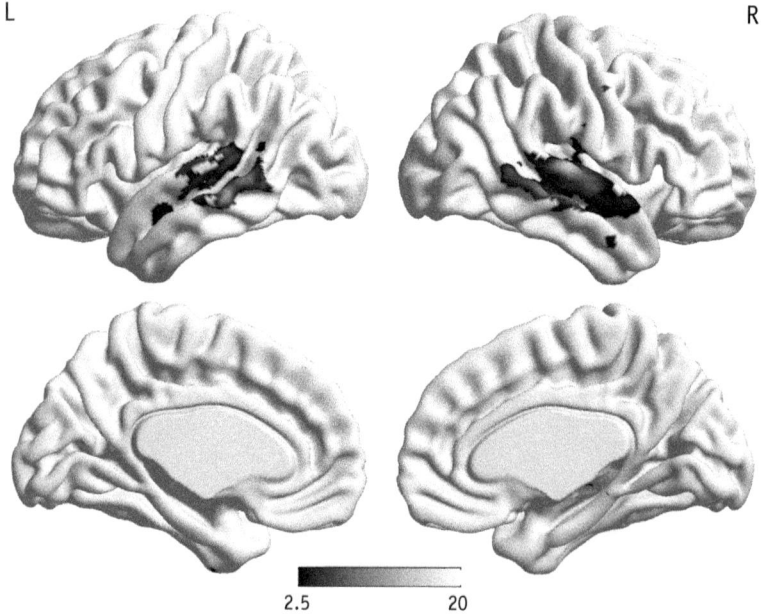

Figure 4.3 fMRI showing only activation of the Heschl's gyrus after voice test in patient with PVS. (Compare this paucity of activation with Figure 4.2)

asking the patient to imagine playing tennis and to imagine walking through their house. Two other fMRI paradigms are asking the patient to try to name objects when looking at a screen, resulting in activation of language areas; and pretending to swim, resulting in activation of premotor cortex.

In recent studies, communication could be established in exceptional patients correlating "yes and no responses" to these above mentioned tasks. ("if you mean yes think you are playing tennis" and so forth). Although yes and no communication seems to exists in MCS, none of these studies in patients with MCS have yet established a reproducible way of communicating with the patient to get a sense of their well-being, agony, or perhaps more likely absence of emotions. A more complex question is whether there is a lack of theory of mind—the ability to perceive different intentions of others.[4] Does this mean there are there patients who signal by fMRI that they are "in there" but cannot use verbal or motor movements to express their needs? This implausible scenario in devastatingly injured patients was challenged by some patient examples where commands could elicit brain activation. Even more, some investigations have found that electromyographic activations may occur—not noticed with clinical observation—after asking to move a hand.[5] Whether fMRI-based communication is possible is currently being investigated.[36,50]

Functional MRI studies into pain perception in MCS also have found intact networks, with cingulate areas activating after high-intensity median nerve stimulation, but whether this justifies analgesics in any patient with MCS is not clear. It is very appropriate to ask what a pain reaction means: whether it is truly pain, or whether it is possible that this patient responded in anticipation of pain but has no pain.[6,59] To attribute pain perception to the ability to demonstrate an activated network involved with pain perception is tantamount to attributing dyspnea to a lung infiltrate or ST elevation to chest pain. Pain perception on MRI is not a provable certainty. Even grimacing to a noxious stimulus may not signify anything.

In the early days EEG has been used to demonstrate vegetative state with often marked abnormalities and variable reactivity.[2] More recently EEG—recording from large numbers (129–257) of channels to improve spatial resolution and sampling—has been tested. It was found that these types of EEG could repeatedly detect—in some patients in PVS—a response after a volitional command. This method is far from perfect, since it could not produce these responses in 3 of 12 controls. Moreover, recent reevaluation of the data suggested a major concern with the validity of this claim.[22] Other techniques to demonstrate cortical activity are through event-related brain potentials.[10] Several paradigms have been developed, including audio with a specified tone, harmonic chords, and spoken word pairs. Transcranial magnetic stimulation combined with electroencephalography was able to differentiate responses in vegetative state from minimally conscious state.[42] All these electrodiagnostic tests may seem simpler (and perhaps cheaper) than fMRI, but these studies have been done by experienced study groups and, therefore, are not available to most physicians and therefore have yet no applicability to practice.

Eric Kandel, a nobel laureate said it well "These days it is easy to get irritated with the exaggerated interpretations of brain imaging—for example, that a single fMRI scan can reveal our innermost feelings—and with inflated claims about our understanding of the biological basis of our higher mental processes."[28] Functional MRI is evolving, but the implications of these studies—there is no point in denying it—could be profound. Many neuroscientists now are ready to accept that in some patients there a somethingness rather than a nothingness. The diagnostic accuracy remains unknown. Most patients are tested because the family wants "closure"; in some patients who are subjected to these tests, the physicians may disagree with families that there is some awareness. Of course, the frequencies of false positives and false negatives of these studies are not known. A false positive result may imply capacity for improvement, but then lead to the family being further discouraged. A false negative result may lead to premature withdrawal of support. An ambiguous study or artifactual study leads to nothing. In this new world of neuroimaging there are a lot of "thought to be's," "appear to be's," and "could be's." The bottom line is that we need hard proof that patients in a prolonged coma or MCS have—or will get—a satisfying quality of life before we attribute practical value to these studies.

In Practice

When does consciousness become impaired, and what is the clinical spectrum of abnormalities? First, there is the ubiquitous drowsy patient and the drowsy and wild patient. Many patients who are "encephalopathic" or "delirious" have an abnormal attention span, cannot perform simple tasks, or cannot remember events. Many of these patients have either an underlying renal or liver disease or are exposed to major side effects of commonly known drugs—not infrequently due to poor clearance of the drug. A delirium is a very common complication in the ICU and follows critical medical or surgical illness—it is most often noted after a major surgical procedure. It may be seen in more than 50% of critically ill patients depending on the severity of the underlying illness, age, and the previous cognitive status of the patient. Delirium in critically ill patients is associated with later cognitive defects but it is unclear if these patients had a poor baseline to begin with. Delirium may be superimposed on a previously undiagnosed dementing illness. Delirium has been associated with reduced brain volumes or confluent white matter changes.

Many patients with ICU delirium do not have pure or even predominant hyperactivity. Instead, mixed and hypoactive forms of delirium are more common. The worst thing one can do is to name it a metabolic encephalopathy and add the adjective "multifactorial." Nonetheless the terms "delirium," "metabolic encephalopathy," and "toxic encephalopathy" remain poor descriptions of acute global nonlocalizing brain dysfunction, often with no good explanation besides the

Table 4.1 **Distinguishing Clinical Features Between PVS and MCS**

Test	PVS	MCS
Eyes	Absent tracking Absent fixating Nystagmoid and roving	Tracking or fixating
Verbal	Absent	Sounds Moans Words
Grimacing	Absent (mostly)	Present
Sounds	Startle	Looks to sound
Movement	Reflex only	Voluntary or localizing

more common causes such as alcohol withdrawal, drug intoxication, drug interactions, sepsis, or a hypertensive urgency. Delirium is common in patients with polypharmacy, which makes pinpointing the culprit nearly impossible. The drugs that should be considered (and thus stopped) are benzodiazepines and opioids, particularly when given in incremental doses. The relationship between sedation and delirium may be oversimplified.[18]

Second, these concepts of wakefulness and awareness can be translated to clinical examination of comatose patients.[56] A careful clinical examination remains key, and the diagnosis of prolonged comatose states is largely descriptive. Eye movements need most attention, because response to tracking objects distinguishes between a PVS (inconsistent or absent), akinetic mutism (no tracking but spontaneous focusing on moving targets), and MCS (tracking always present).[24,25] The major differences between different disorders of consciousness are shown in Table 4.1. The terminology may remain open to debate,[29,57] but there now appears to be some reasonable understanding of what these conditions mean and what characteristics will lead to diagnosis.

The diagnosis of PVS is very uncommon, because most patients in this condition improve or even awaken within three to six months. Therefore, a misdiagnosed PVS may be a recovered PVS. The massive destruction in the cortical layers and thalamus at autopsy, absence of operational modular networks after stimulation when using fMRI, marked reduction in glucose metabolism on PET, and markedly depressed EEG PVS are all test results that confirm a clinical examination showing a nonsapient being. The general rule remains that if the clinical findings of PVS are still present after 3 months in nontraumatic coma (i.e., after anoxic-ischemic injury, hypoglycemia, infections or status epilepticus), substantial recovery is not anticipated. In traumatic brain injury, 12 months are needed for certainty, but recovery to an MCS may nonetheless occur beyond this time limit.

There may be some therapeutic options in patients with impaired consciousness. Treatment of MCS has been of most interest, and now data suggest that amantadine

> **BY THE WAY**
>
> - Delirium can be silent or hyperactive
> - Causes of delirium are often not found
> - Anoxic injury is more damaging than trauma
> - Fluctuation may be due to bithalamic injury
> - Find an explanation even if it requires an MRI
> - Never say the patient will never wake up

> **UNCONSCIOUSNESS BY THE NUMBERS**
>
> - ~100% of patients in PVS are permanent after 2 years
> - ~ 90% of patients in PVS die within 5 years
> - ~ 75% of patients in MCS improve to better functionality
> - ~ 20% of patients in PVS are misdiagnosed or have recovered
> - ~ 10% of fMRI of patients in PVS show activity with tasks
> - ~ 1% of fMRI of patients in PVS may respond to tasks

100 mg twice daily for 2 weeks followed by 150 mg twice daily at week 3 and 200 mg twice daily at week 4 helps with recovery.[21] A zolpidem (10 mg) trial may be considered, but response is variable and mostly absent.[55] Methylphenidate (Ritalin) is a dopaminergic agent that improves processing speed, attention, and possibly memory. Other dopaminergic drugs, selective norepinephrine reuptake inhibitors (atomoxetine), has been considered in postconcussional cognitive impairment, but not in MCS. Others have tried fluoxetine 20 mg daily (selective serotonin reuptake inhibitor) with some effect in motor response.[11]

Interest in deep brain stimulation has rekindled, and bipolar stimulation of thalamic nuclei has been considered with variable results.[44,46] No further data that can be appropriately scrutinized has been forthcoming.

There is little evidence these treatments could produce harm in these human beings. On the other hand, one can see that these patients may become perceived as a "neglected" group of patients, while there truly may not be much offered here that will lead to improved functional outcome. It also remains unexamined whether increased awareness of a major neurologic handicap causes more agony to the patient who is becoming more fully aware of his ordeal when aggressive treatment results in little functional improvement.

Putting It All Together

- Prolonged unconsciousness is very rare
- Awakening may not mean registering events

- Few respond to stimulants
- Certain points of no return exist, beyond which the patient will not likely awaken
- Clinical observation by experts trumps neuroimaging

References

1. Adams JH, Graham DI, Jennett B. The neuropathology of the vegetative state after an acute brain insult. *Brain* 2000;123:1327–1338.
2. Babiloni C, Sarà M, Vecchio F, et al. Cortical sources of resting-state alpha rhythms are abnormal in persistent vegetative state patients. *Clin Neurophysiol* 2009;120:719–729.
3. Balkin TJ, Braun AR, Wesensten NJ, et al. The process of awakening: a PET study of regional brain activity patterns mediating the re-establishment of alertness and consciousness. *Brain* 2002;125:2308–2319.
4. Bekinschtein T, Leiguarda R, Armony J, et al. Emotion processing in the minimally conscious state. *J Neurol Neurosurg Psychiatry* 2004;75:788.
5. Bekinschtein TA, Coleman MR, Niklison J 3rd, Pickard JD, Manes FF. Can electromyography objectively detect voluntary movement in disorders of consciousness? *J Neurol Neurosurg Psychiatry* 2008;79:826–828.
6. Boly M, Faymonville ME, Schnakers C, et al. Perception of pain in the minimally conscious state with PET activation: an observational study. *Lancet Neurol* 2008;7:1013–1020.
7. Boly M, Garrido MI, Gosseries O, et al. Preserved feedforward but impaired top-down processes in the vegetative state. *Science* 2011;332:858–862.
8. Buckner RL, Andrews-Hanna JR, Schacter DL. The brain's default network: anatomy, function, and relevance to disease. *Ann N Y Acad Sci* 2008;1124:1–38.
9. Cairns R. Disturbances of consciousness with lesions of the brainstem and diencephalon. *Brain* 1952;75:109–146.
10. Cavinato M, Freo U, Ori C, et al. Post-acute P300 predicts recovery of consciousness from traumatic vegetative state. *Brain Inj* 2009;23:973–980.
11. Chollet F, Tardy J, Albucher JF, et al. Fluoxetine for motor recovery after acute ischemic stroke (FLAME): a randomised placebo-controlled trial. *Lancet Neurol* 2011;10:123–130.
12. Crone JS, Ladurner G, Höller Y, et al. Deactivation of the default mode network as a marker of impaired consciousness: an fMRI study. *PLoS One* 2011;6:e26373.
13. Cruse D, Chennu S, Chatelle C, et al. Bedside detection of awareness in the vegetative state: a cohort study. *Lancet* 2011;378:2088–2094.
14. Cruse D, Owen A. Consciousness revealed: new insights into the vegetative and minimally conscious states. *Curr Opin Neurol* 2010;23:656–660.
15. Daltrozzo J, Wioland N, Mutschler V, et al. Cortical information processing in coma. *Cogn Behav Neurol* 2009;22:53–62.
16. Di HB, Yu SM, Weng XC, et al. Cerebral response to patient's own name in the vegetative and minimally conscious states. *Neurology* 2007;68:895–899.
17. Fernández-Espejo D, Soddu A, Cruse D, et al. A role for the default network in the bases of disorders of consciousness. *Ann Neurol* 2012;72:335–343.
18. Fraser GL, Worby CP, Riker RR. Dissecting sedation-induced delirium. *Crit Care Med* 2013;41:1144–1146.
19. Giacino JT, Ashwal S, Childs N, et al. The minimally conscious state: definition and diagnostic criteria. *Neurology* 2002;58:349–353.
20. Giacino JT, Kalmar K, Whyte J. The JFK Coma Recovery Scale-Revised: measurement characteristics and diagnostic utility. *Arch Phys Med Rehabil* 2004;85:2020–2029.
21. Giacino JT, Whyte J, Bagiella E, et al. Placebo-controlled trial of amantadine for severe traumatic brain injury. *N Engl J Med* 2012;366:819–826.

22. Goldfine AM, Bardin JC, Noirhomme Q, et al. Reanalysis of "Bedside detection of awareness in the vegetative state: a cohort study." *Lancet* 2013;381:289–291.
23. Ingvar DH, Sourander P. Destruction of the reticular core of the brain stem: a patho-anatomical follow-up of a case of coma of three years' duration. *Arch Neurol* 1970;23:1–8.
24. Jennett B, Plum F. Persistent vegetative state after brain damage. A syndrome in search of a name. *Lancet* 1972;1:734–737.
25. Jennett B. Thirty years of the vegetative state: clinical, ethical and legal problems. *Prog Brain Res* 2005;150:537–543.
26. Jones B. Arousal systems. *Front Biosci* 2003;8:438–451.
27. Pandharipande PP, Girard TD, Jackson JC, et al. Long-term cognitive impairment after critical illness. *N Eng J Med* 2013;369:1306–1316.
28. Kandel E. New Science of Mind. *New York Times*, September 6, 2013.
29. Laureys S, Schiff ND. Coma and consciousness: paradigms (re)framed by neuroimaging. *Neuroimage* 2012;61:478–491.
30. Logothetis NK. What we can do and what we cannot do with fMRI. *Nature* 2008;453:869–878.
31. Logothetis NK, Pauls J, Augath M, Trinath T, Oeltermann A. Neurophysiological investigation of the basis of the fMRI signal. *Nature* 2001;412:150–157.
32. Magoun HW. *The Waking Brain*. Springfield (IL), Charles C. Thomas, 1958.
33. Maquet P. Functional neuroimaging of normal sleep by positron emission tomography. *J Sleep Res* 2000;9:207–231.
34. Monti MM, Laureys S, Owen A. The vegetative state. *BMJ* 2010;341:c3765.
35. Moruzzi G, Magoun H. Brain stem reticular formation and activation of the EEG. *EEG Clin Neurophysiol* 1949;1:455–473.
36. Naci L, Owen AM. Making every word count for vegetative patients. *JAMA Neurology* 2013; in press.
37. Norton L, Hutchison RM, Young GB, et al. Disruptions of functional connectivity in the default mode network of comatose patients. *Neurology* 2012;78:175–181.
38. Parvizi J, Damasio A. Consciousness and the brainstem. *Cognition* 2001;79:135–160.
39. Parvizi J, Damasio AR. Neuroanatomical correlative brainstem coma. *Brain* 2003;126:1524–1536.
40. Raichle ME, Mintun MA. Brain work and brain imaging. *Annu Rev Neurosci* 2006;29:449–476.
41. Ropper AH. Cogito ergo sum by MRI. *N Engl J Med* 2010;382:648–649.
42. Rosanova M, Gosseries O, Casarotto S, et al. Recovery of cortical effective connectivity and recovery of consciousness in vegetative patients. *Brain* 2012;135:1308–1320..
43. Saper C, Chou I, Scammell T. The sleep switch: hypothalamic control of sleep and wakefulness. *Trends Neurosci* 2001;24:726–731.
44. Schiff ND, Giacino JT, Kalmar K, et al. Behavioural improvements with thalamic stimulation after severe traumatic brain injury. *Nature* 2007;448:600–603.
45. Schiff ND, Ribary U, Moreno DR, et al. Residual cerebral activity and behavioural fragments can remain in the persistently vegetative brain. *Brain* 2002;125:1210–1234.
46. Sen AN, Campbell PG, Yadla S, Jallo J, Sharan AD. Deep brain stimulation in the management of disorders of consciousness: a review of physiology, previous reports, and ethical considerations. *Neurosurg Focus* 2010;29:E14.
47. Sharp DJ, Beckmann CF, Greenwood R, et al. Default mode network functional and structural connectivity after traumatic brain injury. *Brain* 2011;134:2233–2247.
48. Silva S, Alacoque X, Fourcade O, et al. Wakefulness and loss of awareness: brain and brainstem interaction in the vegetative state. *Neurology* 2010;74:313–320.
49. Smith P, Samson W, Ferguson A. Cardiovascular actions of orexin-a in the rat subfornical organ. *J Neuroendocrinol* 2007;19:7–13.
50. Sorger B, Dahmen B, Reithler J, et al. Another kind of "BOLD Response": answering multiple-choice questions via online decoded single-trial brain signals. *Prog Brain Res* 2009;177:275–292.

51. Trenell M, Marshall N, Rogers N. Sleep and metabolic control: waking to a problem? *Clin Exp Pharmacol Physiol* 2007;34:1–9.
52. Vanderwolf CH, Stewart DJ. Thalamic control of neocortical activation: a critical re-evaluation. *Brain Res Bull* 1988;20:529–538.
53. Vanhaudenhuyse A, Noirhomme Q, Tshibanda LJ, et al. Default network connectivity reflects the level of consciousness in non-communicative brain-damaged patients. *Brain* 2010;133:161–171.
54. Vogt B, Laureys S. Posterior cingulate, precuneal and retrosplenial cortices: cytology and components of the neural network correlates of consciousness. *Prog Brain Res* 2005;150:205–217.
55. Whyte J, Myers R. Incidence of clinically significant responses to zolpidem among patients with disorders of consciousness: a preliminary placebo controlled trial. *Am J Phys Med Rehabil* 2009;88:410–418
56. Wijdicks EFM. Bare essentials: *Coma Pract Neurol*. 2010;10:51–60.
57. Wijdicks EFM. Being comatose: why definition matters. *Lancet Neurol* 2012;11:657–658.
58. Wijdicks EFM. The Comatose Patient. 2nd edition: Oxford University Press. New York, 2014.
59. Yu T, Lang S, Vogel D et al. Patients with unresponsive wakefulness syndrome respond to the pain cries of other people. *Neurology* 2013:80:345–352.
60. Zhang D, Raichle ME. Disease and the brain's dark energy. *Nat Rev Neurol* 2010;6:15–28.

5

Neurology of Breathing

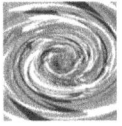

For starters: respiratory failure and shortness of breath is not ordinarily due to a neurologic disorder. Respiratory failure is far more common—at least in the hospital and general ICU—due to diastolic heart failure and acute exacerbation of chronic obstructive pulmonary disease. Respiratory failure is uncommon in acute neuromucular disease and more common in established progressive disease. It should come as a surprise if it is the first manifestation of acute neuromucular disease. It is a completely a different story with acute brain injury. In fact without resuscitation patients with catastrophic brain injury die from respiratory arrest and not cardiac arrest.

As a general rule the airway and breathing—with a few exceptions—can rapidly become abnormal in acute brain injury. The A and B in the ABC of first aid are so important in acute neurologic disease that it almost seems invented for that purpose. Insofar as it can be urgently assessed, compromised breathing in patients with acute neurologic disease is often due to oropharyngeal collapse, aspiration, poor respiratory drive, or pulmonary mechanics—all of that leads to poor gas exchange or ventilation.

It is not an easy task for physicians to find out why this particular acutely ill neurologic patient under these particular circumstances breathes this way, and it is even more daunting when a ventilated patient is struggling. Furthermore, breathing difficulties in a setting of acute neurologic disease is so fundamentally different from that in patients with pulmonary disease that a good understanding of its pathophysiology should be part of core knowledge. In other words, what are neurologic breathing patterns, and how specific are they? What changes physiologically when respiratory failure is associated with weakness of the respiratory muscles? Are there quantifiable criteria for assisting with mechanical ventilation?

There is a good reason for physicians to regard breathing in acute neurologic disease as important and a neurologic examination is incomplete without an assessment of breathing. This chapter attempts to explain the logic of this complex physiology and all that goes with it.

Principles

Breathing involves ventilation (gas exchange in the lung) and respiration (inhalation and exhalation). Ventilation requires room air (21% oxygen or more) and clearance of carbon dioxide. Respiration requires a generator.

CENTRAL COMPONENT OF BREATHING

To begin with, breathing is generated but also coordinated in the medulla oblongata. This is essentially a neural oscillator system and it begins to function in utero. Fetal respiratory movements of the diaphragm coincide with the start of this oscillator—the pre-Bötzinger complex—and main generator of breathing. It is the only group of medulla oblongata neurons whose inactivation results in complete apnea. There may be another oscillator—the epF or neurons next to the VII nucleus—which is possibly the ancient rhythm generator in aquatic vertebrates. The pre-Bötzinger complex represents the newer oscillator that emerged with the evolution of the lung and its complement of muscles.

Breathing is automatic (involuntary), and we do not think about it unless we become breathless.[12,14] We can override this oscillator temporarily when we yawn, sneeze, cough, laugh, and cry, all with a stereotyped breathing pattern. We can also voluntarily hold our breath or hyperventilate. As we will see later, certain lesions will prevent some of these actions.

There are several main systems involved in breathing, which involves the motor and sensory cortex.[5,12] Awareness of changes in respiration and ability to sense discomfort are likely located in areas involved with awareness of body and emotions. The insula and operculum mediate dyspnea, and the cingulate gyrus, prefrontal cortex, and supramarginal gyrus integrate emotional and sensory aspects of respiration. The role of the cortex is likely minimal, but it is able to detect a sensation of breathlessness—when associated with elevated $PaCO_2$, it activates the limbic system and parietal cortex.[4,7,22]

Most of the breathing apparatus is in the medulla oblongata and pons, which send signals to the respiratory muscles. There is feedback from sensors including central and peripheral chemoreceptors and pulmonary mechanoreceptors, which relay information to the respiratory control center.

The autonomic rhythm of breathing is located in the ventral respiratory group (VRG) ventral to the nucleus ambiguus in the medulla oblongata (Figure 5.1). There is a cell population for each specific function. Within this complex is the pre-Bötzinger region, mentioned before, which is likely the main respiratory rhythm generator.

The VRG contains inspiratory (rostrally placed) and expiratory (caudally placed) neurons; the function of these neurons is to drive not only the spinal respiratory neurons innervating the intercostal and abdominal muscles but also the upper airway muscles of inspiration. This explains why acute brainstem lesions not only involve respiratory rhythm but also cause great difficulty with maintaining an upper airway.

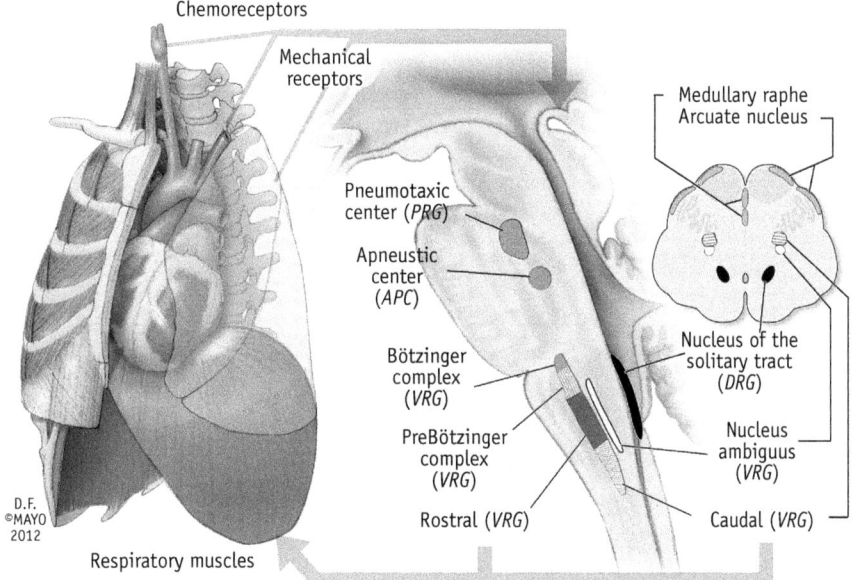

Figure 5.1 Central control of breathing and feedback (VRG, ventral respiratory group; PRG, pontine respiratory group; APC, apneustic center; DRG, dorsal respiratory group).

Another group in the medulla oblongata, the dorsal respiratory group (DRG), is composed of cells in the nucleus tractus solitarius and is in the dorsal medial region of the medulla oblongata. The DRG is responsible for inspiration. The DRG receives fibers from cranial nerves IX and X, which provide information about PO_2, PCO_2, and pH from the peripheral chemoreceptors. The vagus nerve provides information about the pulmonary mechanics via pulmonary mechanoreceptors. This is not a major feedback system, which became apparent after denervated lung transplantations.

Two areas in the pons also play a role in respiratory control. First, a pontine respiratory group (PRG) is situated in the upper pons; this center regulates termination of inspiration. When inspiration shortens, the respiratory rate increases. The PRG regulates tidal volume and respiratory rate, and its function, therefore, involves adjusting or calibrating rather than generating breaths. In addition, animal experiments have identified an apneustic center (APC) located in the lower pons. If this area is lesioned, it will produce inspiratory gasps, possibly because the medullary respiratory neurons are now without a control mechanism. Clinically, this is seen in moribund patients with secondary brainstem injury who breathe inspiratory gasps before an apnea.

How is respiration further regulated? Mostly through changes in PCO_2, PO_2, and pH of the arterial blood[8,10,21,22] and, to a much lesser degree, through input from lung parenchyma receptors. These specialized receptors respond to mechanical stimulation (stretch reflexes) and transmit their input through unmyelinated vagus nerve fibers. This may also be a mechanism that creates a sensation of dyspnea and altered ventilatory pattern in patients with pulmonary edema, although hypoxemia is a far more likely mechanism in general. The arterial PCO_2 and PO_2 are dependent on several components, as shown in Figure 5.2.

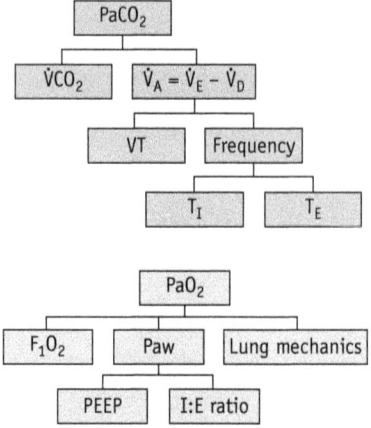

Figure 5.2 Factors determining PaO_2 and $PaCO_2$.
$\dot{V}CO_2$, carbon dioxide production; V_A, alveolar volume; V_E, expired volume; VD, deadspace; V_T, tidal volume; T_I, inspiratory time; T_E, expiratory time, F_IO_2, fraction of inspired oxygen; P_{aw}, positive airway pressure; PEEP, positive end expiratory pressure; I, inspiratory; E, expiratory.

Both hypercapnia and hypoxemia significantly increase stimulation of chemoreceptors—anatomically separate receptors that are located on the ventrolateral surface of the medulla (Figure 5.1). These chemoreceptors sense the pH of the extracellular fluid and basically the pH of the CSF. Because of the characteristics of the blood-brain barrier—which is impermeable to hydrogen and HCO_3 ions—the PCO_2 in CSF is equal to the arterial PCO_2. (Strictly speaking, due to carbon dioxide production from neurons, the PCO_2 in CSF is 10 mm Hg higher than arterial PCO_2.) According to the Henderson-Hasselbach equation, an increase in PCO_2 results in a decrease in pH. Therefore, an increase in arterial PCO_2 results in an increase in CSF PCO_2 and a decrease in CSF pH. This decrease in CSF pH stimulates the central chemoreceptors; this results in an increase in ventilation. Hyperventilation, in turn, reduces arterial PCO_2, and because the mechanism just described reduces the CSF pH, it is important to mention here that changes in arterial pH may take much longer because hydrogen ions cross the blood-brain barrier too slowly to affect the central chemoreceptors. In other words, there is acidotic stimulation of the peripheral chemoreceptors, and arterial PCO_2 falls through feedback hyperventilation. This then results in diffusion of CO_2 out of CSF, an increase in CSF pH, and a decrease in central chemoreceptor stimulation. However, several hours are necessary before this occurs. In addition, there are peripheral chemoreceptors that are located in the carotid bodies and the aortic bodies and are usually close to the bifurcation of the common carotid artery.

Usually ventilation is stimulated after PO_2 is less than 60 mm Hg. The afferent nerve from the carotid body increases its traffic when there is a decrease in arterial PO_2, decrease in arterial pH, hypoperfusion, hyperthermia, and certain drugs (e.g., doxapram) that stimulate respiration through the peripheral chemoreceptors.

The relationship between PO_2 and PCO_2 is complex. When arterial PCO_2 is increased, ventilation increases despite a normal PaO_2.

PERIPHERAL COMPONENT OF BREATHING

Lungs, phrenic nerve, respiratory muscles, and the chest wall are all part of another major component of breathing. The main muscle is the diaphragm. All respiratory muscles act in concert during abnormal breathing, but most are silent under normal breathing conditions.

Normal quiet breathing is largely accomplished by contraction of the diaphragm. In general, the diaphragm is responsible for approximately two-thirds of the ventilatory effort to generate inspiration. It may be supplemented by accessory inspiratory muscles including the intercostals, scalene, and sternocleidomastoid muscles. Expiration is mostly due to recoil of the thoracic cage, but abdominal muscles are also necessary to generate expiration and are responsible for a forceful cough. The diaphragm is a large muscle and necessary to significantly increase lung volume. The innervation of the diaphragm is by the phrenic nerves that branch from C_3-C_5. The respiratory load, an important determinant, is dependent on the sum of resistance of inspiratory flow, the resistance of the chest wall and lungs, and the positive pressure at peak expiration. When inspiratory muscles contract, a negative force overcomes this respiratory load, resulting in inward movement of air. With weakness, the respiratory load can only be partly overcome, leading to less airflow and collapse of lung areas. This collapse leads to shunting and hypoxemia. Hypoxemia will stimulate the respiratory centers as explained earlier, but it will not generate better long volumes; hence we see rapid shallow breathing. The consequences of neuromuscular respiratory failure and its management is discussed in detail in another volume (handling difficult situations) in this series.

In Practice

So, is all this information relevant to clinical practice? Yes, to some degree. There are three circumstances in which this fundamental knowledge is necessary.

THE ABNORMALLY BREATHING ACUTELY ILL NEUROLOGIC PATIENT (CENTRAL CAUSES)

The most common question neurologists should ask themselves is whether the patient has a neurologic origin of breathing problems. These are patients who have developed marked hypoxemic hypercapnic respiratory failure, had documented apneic episodes, periodic breathing, and generally are unweanable from the mechanical ventilator. Usually very circumscript lesions such as small hemorrhages, infarcts, or multiple sclerosis plaques in the brainstem may cause interruptions in pathways.[14] Ischemic stroke in the brainstem—involving the tractus solitarius—nucleus ambiguus, and nucleus retroambiguus have also been associated with apnea and failure to respond to increase in $PaCO_2$. Sleep apnea can be found in many patients with a stroke and is usually part of the premorbid condition.

Abnormalities in respiratory patterns are paroxysm of hyperventilation, apneustic breathing, nocturnal sleep apnea, and inability to voluntarily change pattern of respiration (unable to cough or hold breath). Respiration (and oxygenation) also changes with seizures (any type) and may cause apnea.[2,3,16,20]

Table 5.1 summarizes the breathing patterns in acute neurologic disease. There are several patterns, but in clinical practice there are quite a few confounders. These include sedatives such as propofol muting the drive, and opioids reducing the drive and causing hypoventilation with apneic pauses.[24] Furthermore, compensation for hypoxemia will increase respiratory drive, and irregular breathing may be simply intermittent upper airway obstruction.

The breathing pattern known as Biot's respiration (ataxic respiration) is irregular with changing tidal volumes and rapid with intermittent pauses. It is often confused with cluster breathing, which is regular with identical tidal volumes and with pauses in between. Biot breathing can be contrasted with Cheyne-Stokes breathing (periodic stereotypical crescendo-decrescendo hyperpnea followed by apnea) and apneustic breathing (periodic prolonged inspiratory hold).

Central neurogenic hyperventilation (CNH) can be seen in comatose patients with anoxic-ischemic encephalopathy and in patients with upper brainstem

Table 5.1 **Respiratory Abnormalities with Acute Brain Injury**

Site	Abnormality
Medulla oblongata (arcuate nucleus)	Hypoventilation, apneic spells
Medulla oblongata (tegmentum)	Sleep apnea (obstructive)
Medulla oblongata (nucleus tractus solitarius)	Hypoxemia from massive pulmonary edema
Medulla oblongata (nucleus ambiguus)	Apnea during drowsiness and sleep (Ondine's curse)
Medulla oblongata (dorsomedial area)	Ataxic breathing
Pons (midbrain)	Central neurogenic hyperventilation
Pons (caudal)	Apneustic (inspiratory cramp breathing)
Cortex	Periodic breathing (cluster, Cheyne-Stokes)

compression and shift from a new hemispheric lesion. The disorder is also a consequence of a midbrain or pontine lesion and can be associated with pontine hemorrhages, embolus to the basilar artery, and progressive signs of brainstem compression from a cerebellar lesion. For unknown reasons, the incidence of primary brainstem lymphoma or astrocytoma in patients with central neurogenic hyperventilation is high. Infiltration of tumor, whether lymphoma or astrocytoma, presumably destroys the inhibiting descending neurons from the pons to the medullary respiratory center. CNH has also been reported in multiple sclerosis and brainstem encephalitis; but again, the responsible lesion is in the pons. The patient cannot inhibit respiratory drive.

In traumatic brain injury, periodic hyperventilation may occur with tachycardia, fever, and sweating and is related to sympathetic hyperactivity syndrome. It may be the most commonly underrecognized manifestation of acute brain injury and thus the most commonly undertreated. CNH is usually continuously present and seemingly wears out the patient. Hyperventilation in this setting can also be more erratic and may result in difficulty ventilating patients due to asynchrony with the ventilator. In sustained neurogenic hyperventilation, respiratory alkalosis is considerable, with pH values greater than 7.6. This type of breathing disorder is best muted with infusion of potent respiratory depressants such as fentanyl.

The term "Ondine's curse" has been used in hypoventilation syndrome and loss of automatic ventilation. Pulmonary pathology must be excluded if there is a rise in PCO_2 and no response in ventilation. The condition can be easily mimicked by high doses of opioids. Acquired forms of Ondine's curse have always involved lesions in the respiratory centers of the medulla oblongata. Multiple cases of central hypoventilation have been described with acute stroke, tumors, infections, multiple sclerosis, and cervical cordotomy. Treatment of Ondine's curse is BiPAP with a back up rate but all patients need a sleep study to look for obstructive component. Next step is the tracheostomy with long term ventilation. Diaphragmatic pacing is rarely needed except in congenital forms.

Of all "neurogenic" breathing patterns, Cheyne-Stokes breathing is not only the best known but also the least noted or documented. Cheyne-Stokes breathing is most often seen in sleep and commonly seen with central sleep apnea. Central sleep apnea as a consequence of acute stroke is very common and has been reported in up to 50% of patients with both hemispheric and brainstem strokes. Hypercapnea and hypoxemia occur during sleep, and there is no evidence of upper airway obstruction.

THE ABNORMALLY BREATHING ACUTELY ILL NEUROLOGIC PATIENT (PERIPHERAL CAUSES)

There are a few important pieces of information to keep in mind. When the diaphragm is nonfunctioning, the accessory muscles can compensate; however, failure of the diaphragm to adequately contract will result in a decrease of the functional residual capacity of the lungs, little peripheral alveolar recruitment that will then result in no ventilation but still adequate perfusion, also known as shunting. This will then result in hypoxemia, further stimulating the chemoreceptors and in turn resulting in increased respiratory frequency, but without increase in tidal volume.

In peripheral neurologic disorders, whether acute or chronic, most of the time there is presence of oropharyngeal weakness in a patient with respiratory weakness. This combination of oropharyngeal weakness and neuromuscular weakness places the patient at immediate risk, from inability to clear secretions and upper airway obstruction and inability to oxygenate. In some instances, the main innervating nerve—the phrenic nerve—is involved, mostly from autoimmune neuropathy, local trauma, or an invasive mass. One phrenic nerve dysfunction can easily be compensated for; involvement of both phrenic nerves is also compensated for, but dyspnea occurs with exertion or change to supine position. Lack of movement of one side of the diaphragm is found on thoracic ultrasound (descending diaphragm moves toward the probe in normal aspiration).

Acute spinal cord injury may impact on breathing almost immediately when the lesion is at C3 or higher and permanent. Patients with high cervical cord lesions also have airway hyperreactivity. Abdominal strapping is necessary in many patients because the abdominal muscles are paralyzed.

Diaphragmatic function can be assessed clinically. Vital capacity is a function that can be assessed at the bedside. A mouthpiece is placed, and the patient is asked to exhale after maximal inhalation. Typically, a vital capacity may already change with a change in position. A decrease in vital capacity of approximately 20% with position change from a sitting to a lying position is indicative of failing mechanics. The maximal inspiratory pressures are a measure of diaphragmatic function, while the maximal expiratory pressure is largely a measure of abdominal muscle. Maximal inspiratory and expiratory pressures can also be measured via a mouthpiece and spirometer at the bedside. Alternatively a sniff nasal inspiratory pressure can be checked. Again, a peak flow meter does not measure these abnormalities, and they may indicate only strength of coughing and not respiratory function. Pulmonary function tests may also be unreliable because patients may suck in cheek muscles and such a maneuver should be noted by the physician.

Chest X-ray is important because it may suggest a diaphragm elevation, atelectasis due to poor alveolar recruitment, or earlier signs of aspiration. Arterial blood gases are not always helpful, as hypoxemia has already been noted with a pulse oximeter. The presence of increased $PaCO_2$ and bicarbonate with a normal pH often indicates chronic hypoventilation.

BASIC SUPPORT OF THE BREATHLESS PATIENT

Most patients require oxygen administration. Oxygen administration is divided into low-flow and high-flow devices. A nasal cannula is a typical example of a low-flow device: the patient receives flow of 100% oxygen at 0–6 L/min. None of the 100% oxygen will eventually reach the alveoli in that pure form, as it is mixed with air in the room (air is normally 0.21 FiO_2). Generally, oxygen delivered by nasal prongs will be an FiO_2 of 0.24 at 1 L/min and may increase up to 0.40 at 5–6 L/min. Each liter of oxygen provides 4% of oxygen starting at 24% (one liter per minute will provide 24%, 2 L will provide 28%, 3 L will provide 32%, and so on). A simple oxygen mask is the next step when higher FiO_2 is necessary. This mask covers the nose and mouth and provides an oxygen reservoir of 100–200 mL at inspiration. Using high flow, FiO_2 can reach 0.8, but usually the FiO_2 will be between 0.32 and 0.6, and the flow is between 5 and 10 L/min (flows less than 5 L/min will result in rebreathing CO_2). The flow can also be increased by using a partial rebreathing mask, which is a mask with an additional 300–600 cc reservoir bag. The oxygen flow will have to keep the bag inflated to inspiration, and about 8–15 L/min can produce an FiO_2 between 0.4 and 0.7. With inspiration, the patient inhales 100% from the reservoir bag. The idea here is that exhaled gas that enters the reservoir bag is high in oxygen because it is coming from the uppermost parts of the airway. In a nonrebreather mask, the flow must be high enough to prevent full collapse of the reservoir bag during inhalation and more than 12 L/min is required.

Hypoxemia is usually detected by changes in the patient resulting in restlessness, tachycardia or bradycardia, tachypnea, and in the extreme, cyanosis. Failure to correct hypoxemia with oxygen administration should prompt mechanical (noninvasive or invasive) support of ventilation.

The decision to intubate remains clinical but can be made based on the following criteria: inability to cough up secretions, tachypnea, hemodynamic instability, and abnormal arterial blood gas with abnormal $PaCO_2$ or PaO_2. There are other, less subtle signs: anxiety, sternocleidomastoid muscle contractions, grunting, nasal flaring (contraction of dilator muscle of external nares), mouth opening, and with rising $PaCO_2$ increasing drowsiness.

THE MECHANICALLY VENTILATED PATIENT

Neurologists walking into the emergency room or intensive care unit most often see a patient on a mechanical ventilator. The decision to assist the patient with ventilation often has been made earlier, and now crucial questions are: Is the patient adequately ventilated and oxygenated? Is the patient tolerating the ventilator or still fighting it? Is there evidence that mechanical ventilation is improving the clinical condition?

Here is some information that is immediately useful and does not require sophisticated knowledge of machinery or pulmonary physiology during mechanical ventilation. There is an array of mechanical ventilators, with new modes introduced with every new model but this is beyond the scope of this chapter and can be found elsewhere.[15,25]

Many patients with neurologic disease and neuromuscular respiratory failure are on a bilevel noninvasive positive airway pressure (BiPAP) ventilation device. There are several areas that need immediate attention. It may be good to assess whether the patient is sitting at a 30-degree angle. Patients with an neuromuscular respiratory failure will breathe much better in a sitting upright position due to absent abdominal compression. The mask should fit well and be comfortable. In a large portion of patients, noninvasive mechanical ventilation is not tolerated when the mask is too tight (two fingers should be allowed between the straps, and tubing to the ventilator should be intact).

Most noninvasive ventilators involve pressure-support ventilation that provides a preset inspiratory pressure to assist in spontaneous breathing efforts. Many ventilators also provide pressure-control ventilation that provides time cycles of preset inspiratory and expiratory pressures and even adjustable inspiratory and expiratory ratios. Additional modes could permit the patient to trigger, and there can be a backup rate. Generally, the difference between peak inspiratory and expiratory positive airway pressures (IPAP and EPAP) is the level of pressure support. For the vast majority of patients with neuromuscular disease, EPAP of 5 cm of water and IPAP of 12 to 14 cm of water is sufficient to improve the condition of the patient. This will then result in a pressure support of about 10 cm of water. A backup rate should be set at 12 to 16 breaths per minute.[20] The spontaneous BiPAP triggering mode is usually set with low pressure volumes. Usually, inspiratory pressure is gradually increased to 10 to 20 cm of water or the tidal volume is increased to 10 to 15 mL/kg to improve respiratory rate, increase the tidal volume, and eventually improve the breathlessness of the patient. Oxygen saturation should be consistently above 90%. If the patient is not tolerating such assisted ventilation, an additional dose of lorazepam 0.5 mg or intravenous dexmethomedine in a low dose (0.2 mcg/kg/hour) could be very helpful in improving machine acceptance by the patient. Arterial blood gases are necessary to monitor the decrease in $PaCO_2$ and increase in PaO_2 as markers of adequate ventilation. Indications for noninvasive ventilation can also be gas exchange abnormalities when the PCO_2 is more than 45 mm Hg, the pH less than 7.35, or the PaO_2/FiO_2 less than 200.

BiPAP is useful for patients with amyotrophic lateral sclerosis and myasthenia gravis and chronic muscular disorders (such as autoimmune necrotic myopathy evolving over years). It is a very unreliable support mode in Guillain-Barré syndrome because the diaphragmatic failure is often too severe to be treated with pressure support alone, and many patients continue to use assessor muscles despite being on BiPAP.

Arriving at the bedside of a patient who has been intubated and is on a mechanical ventilator requires a number of quick checks. First is to exclude retained neuromuscular blockers after intubation. Adequate reversal is with 4 cc glycopyrrolate and 4 mg neostigmine—the 4-4 rule.

The next step is to look at the work of breathing. It is important to observe when the patient is working hard. Is there any sternal retraction? Is the patient moving the diaphragm well or working hard? Is the patient looking anxious or grimacing?

It is important at this point to have a look at the mode of ventilation, whether the patient is on CPAP (continuous positive airway pressure) or SIMV (synchronized intermittent mandatory ventilation) (Figure 5.3).

Then it is important to look specifically at the respiratory rate of the monitor compared to the set respiratory rate. Any discrepancies are problematic. Patients in distress are often tachypenic at 35 per minute.

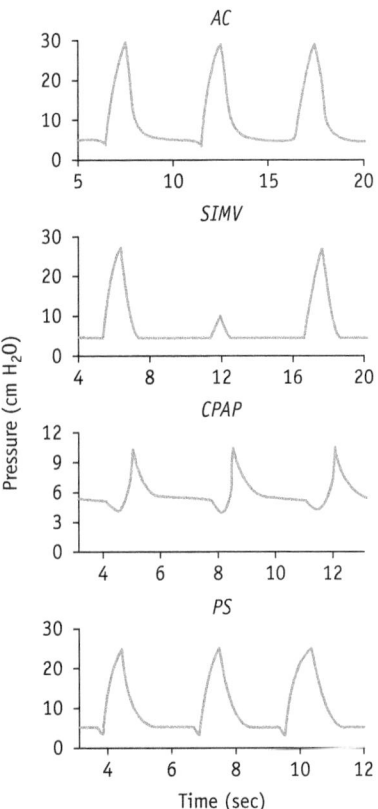

Figure 5.3 Common modes of mechanical ventilation. *AC* (assist control). The first two breaths are patient-triggered, as evidenced by a brief negative deflection in airway pressure followed by a machine-triggered breath. *SIMV* (synchronized intermittent mandatory ventilation). Two machne-triggered breaths have a spontaneous breath in between. *CPAP* (continuous positive airway pressure). All breaths are patient-initiated. *PS* (pressure support). All breaths are patient-initiated. The waveforms of the volume and flow may vary with each breath but have a common rectangular shape.

The tidal volume should be evaluated next. Is the patient generating good tidal volumes commensurate to the amount of pressure support? For example, a 500-mL tidal volume should correspond with pressure support of 10 cm of water. Simply dropping the pressure support to 5 cm of water should reduce the tidal volume by 50%. If less, then it means that the patient might need higher pressure support or a rest period on a set rate.

After the respiratory rate is investigated, the minute ventilation is investigated. Normally minute ventilation is 6–7 liters/minute. Increased minute ventilation indicates hyperventilation and in addition a rapid shallow breathing index can be calculated. This is the ratio of respiratory rate divided by tidal volume and ideally should be less than 100.

Next, the peak pressure is evaluated and should be less than 30 cm of water. Peak plateau pressure is far more complicated to evaluate, but the peak pressure gives sufficient information. If the peak pressure is increased, then this might indicate developing acute respiratory distress syndrome or poor compliance of the lung.

After these simple evaluations, which can be obtained in a matter of seconds, it is important to put a stethoscope to the patient and to listen for adequacy of air movement. The tube placement needs to be verified; normally from lip to tip is 20–25 cm in males and 18–22 cm in females. If the tube "looks" too superficial or too deep, then the chest X-ray can be used for confirmation.

It is also important to have a certain approach if the patient's breathing is labored. This is usually a patient with increased frequency of breathing who seems in major discomfort, with biting on the tube and grimacing. The patient's ventilator dyssynchrony can be solved by briefly bagging the patient. If the patient is bagged, one can feel whether the resistance is increased because of poor compliance. When air is not moving well, this may imply the presence of bronchospasm, air hunger, or even a mucous block.

Another often-asked and important question is whether the ventilator mode is appropriate for the patient. The patient might be overbreathing, which may be very uncomfortable for the patient. Generally, if the patient is not sedated, it is good to change the mode, going from assist-control (AC) to an SIMV of 16 and then moving to an SIMV of 4 and CPAP of 5. If that is tolerated by the patient and other criteria are met, the patient can be extubated.

The parameters shown in Table 5.2 are necessary to assess the adequacy of mechanical ventilation.[4,18,25] There are volume-targeted modes and pressure-targeted modes. In a volume-targeted mode, typically the tidal volume is at 600 mL and the respiratory rate at 10, delivering a minute volume of 6 L/min. The sensitivity is set at –2 cm of water so that the patient can trigger the machine breath. However, if the flow rate does not match inspiratory efforts, the patient can experience shortness of breath, anxiety, and agitation. Adjustment of an appropriate flow rate may improve the breathing comfort. If the patient inspires quickly or more vigorously, various flow rates may match changing inspiratory

Table 5.2 **Ventilator Parameters**

- *Fraction of inspired oxygen (FiO$_2$).* Concentration of oxygen in the inspired gas, usually varying from 0.21 with room air to 1.0 or 100%.
- *Tidal volume (VT).* The volume of gas during a breath usually set at 6 mL/kg to prevent ventilator-associated lunge distention.
- *Respiratory rate or frequency.* The number of breaths per minute that the ventilator delivers. Typically between 10 and 20 breaths per minute.
- *Minute ventilation or VE.* The average volume of gas entering or leaving the lungs per minute, expressed in liters per minute. It is the product of tidal volume × respiratory rate. The minute ventilation is typically between 5 and 10 liters per minute.
- *Peak flow rate or peak inspiratory flow.* The highest flow that is set to deliver the vital capacity during inspiration. With high flows, the speed of gas delivery is faster and the inspiratory time is shorter.
- *Inspiratory and expiratory time and I:E ratio.* This is the speed at which the peak tidal volume is delivered. Normally, the ratio is 1:2 or 1:3.
- *Peak airway pressure.* The total pressure that is necessary to deliver the tidal volume. It is dependent on the airway resistance, lung compliance, and chest wall factors. It is expressed in cm of water.
- *Plateau pressure.* Pressure needed to distend the lung, which can be measured by applying an inspiratory pause setting on the ventilator. It is expressed in cm of water.
- *Sensitivity or trigger sensitivity.* The effort of the patient or negative pressure to trigger a machine breath. Usually it is set at -1 to -2 cm of water, which allows easy triggering. Many ventilators are flow triggering. Some are pressure triggering. The patient makes a spontaneous effort and triggers the machine to deliver the breath.
- *Positive end expiratory pressure, PEEP.* The amount of positive pressure maintained at the end of expiration. Usually also in cm of water. PEEP is used to increase end expiratory lung volume and reduce airspace closure at end expiration.
- *Continuous positive airway pressure, CPAP.* Continuous pressurization of the breathing circuit when a patient breathes spontaneously.
- *Mandatory breath.* The breath in which the timing or size of the breath is completely controlled by the ventilator. Machine triggers or cycles the breath.
- *Spontaneous breath.* The breath in which the timing and size are controlled by the patient.

"Data from references 15, 18, and 25"

demand or may be insufficient. It may be necessary to readjust pressure support and inspiratory and expiratory time setting.

The advantage with the commonly used SIMV plus pressure support is that mandatory breaths are volume targeted and spontaneous breaths are pressure targeted. The patient receives a preset number of volume-targeted mandatory breaths; between these breaths, the patient can breathe spontaneously on pressure-supported breaths. The pressure support is usually sufficient to overcome the airway resistance. If the patient is not taking spontaneous breaths while on a low SIMV rate, the SIMV rate needs to be increased or switched to a full support mode.

CPAP provides a continuous level of positive airway pressure during the respiratory cycle. The ventilator does not provide breaths. The patient initiates all breaths. If the patient is on a CPAP of 5 cm of water, 5 cm of positive pressure is applied on inspiration and expiration. Usually, the application of positive pressure to the airways to keep the alveoli open and prevent closure during expiration is a common weaning mode. There are several factors that increase airway resistance and decrease compliance, including biting down on the tube, obstruction of the endotracheal tube, coughing, the presence of profuse secretions, and a significantly increased respiratory rate. There are also primary pulmonary problem factors that decrease lung compliance, such as pulmonary edema, pneumonia, atelectasis, and endotracheal tube displacement in pneumothorax. Other factors that are outside the pulmonary realm are abdominal contractions on expiration, increased abdominal pressure against the diaphragm due to obesity, ascites or gas distension, shivering, or seizures and a chest wall injury.

Anxiety plays a major role in adjustment of a patient to the ventilator, particularly in patients with an acute peripheral neurologic disorder. Anxiety will increase respiratory rate, increase work of breathing, and increase oxygen requirements; then eventually decompensation and tiring out will cause an increase in PCO_2, a decrease in PO_2, shortness of breath, and further worsening of these events.

It is therefore important to assess patient ventilator interactions that can lead to asynchrony. Synchronous interaction is when the ventilator flow is in phase with the patient effort. Asynchrony is defined as a patient bucking at the ventilator, but often there is also increased work of breathing and increased oxygen requirement. The various forms asynchrony can take have been defined as trigger asynchrony, flow asynchrony, cycle asynchrony, and mode asynchrony. Trigger asynchrony is when the patient is not triggering a ventilator, or the ventilator triggers itself. Usually an insensitive trigger setting on the ventilator is the cause, but respiratory muscle weakness can also reduce triggering of the ventilator. The most common cause, however, is auto-PEEP in patients with obstructive airway disease. This can be remediated by lowering the minute ventilation, shortening the I:E ratio, or improving airway obstruction using mucolytics and bronchodilators. Autotriggering occurs when the ventilator responds to cardiac oscillation or excessive water condensation in the circuit or even a leak in the circuit. Flow asynchrony occurs when the ventilator does not meet the patient inspiratory flow demands. Typically the pressure waveform of each breath differs from each other breath. There is variability both from breath to breath and of the peak airway pressure. This is also detected by comparing the patient-triggered breaths with the breath delivered by manual breath control. A vigorous patient effort may move the airway pressure graphic downward. Usually, also, the patient is tachypneic, has retractions, and chest/abdominal paradox. Treatment involves flow change, either by changing the inspiratory setting, by switching from volume-controlled ventilation to pressure-controlled ventilation, or by increasing the pressure setting or rise time.

Cycle asynchrony occurs if the inspiratory time is too short. In this situation, the patient may double trigger the ventilator. This causes breath stacking, which means that the patient is getting a total volume that is twice what is set. Mode asynchrony occurs when the ventilator delivers different breath types. In general, total volume should never exceed 10 mL/kg and the plateau pressure should be less than 30 cm of water. A lower level of PEEP <10 cm of water may be important to prevent atelectasis, but higher PEEPs, although enabling better compliance and better oxygenation, can lead to ventilator-associated lung injury. A list of common concerns with ventilator management is shown in Table 5.3.

Timing of tracheostomy remains unclear and there is a tendency to move more quickly (to allow dismissal from unit to long term care) and using bedside methods (percutaneous dilatational tracheostomy). It is however a good clinical practice to wait for 10 days unless there is a need for long term protection (facial trauma, prolonged deep coma).

Criteria to assess the readiness of ventilator liberation will involve evidence that respiratory failure is reversed or improved and that there is adequate oxygenation, which is typically defined as a PaO_2 to FiO_2 ratio of more than 200, a PEEP between 5 and 8 cm of water, an FiO_2 that is less than 0.4, and a pH that is normal. There should also be hemodynamic stability, and patients should require no vasopressor therapy or only very low-dose vasopressors. Obviously the patient should be able to initiate a good inspiratory effort and cough. Often it starts with a spontaneous T-piece breathing trial of 1 hour; if that fails, the cause should be determined. If the patient has a spontaneous breathing trial without any difficulties, the aspiration risk, ability to clear secretion, and ability to keep the airway open need to be assessed before extubation. Inflammation and edema may be present, and a quick test for presence of a leak around the cuff with the cuff down may indicate absence of laryngeal edema—the test is far from perfect. The work of breathing may be substantial after extubation, and even a pressure support of 5 cm water—the so-called minimal setting to overcome the resistance of the tube—may reduce work of breathing by approximately 30%. This support would be lost with extubation, and patients may become rapidly tachypneic and hypoxemic.[26]

Finally, another issue in practice is to determine permanent apnea, usually in the setting of a brain death examination. Apnea assessment in mechanically ventilated patients is notoriously unhelpful, and no breathing drive whatsoever can easily be produced with a high-frequency setting (the patient cannot breathe on top of that) or a patient with severe respiratory alkalosis—causing "posthyperventilation

Table 5.3 **Ventilator Alarms**

Alarm Problem	Causes	Interventions
High Pressure	• Blocked or kinked tube, other increased airway resistance or decreased lung compliance, attempting to speak	• Suction secretions • Ensure water condensation from tubing does not drain into patient's airway • Prevent tube movement during turning patient
Continuous high pressure	• Biting down on orally placed tube resulting in peak airway pressure alarm, potential for decreased tidal volume delivery	• Administer bronchodilators • Use tube-securing method with bite block if needed
Low exhaled tidal volume	• Cuff leak • Air leaks due to loose, ventilator circuit or nebulizer connections	• Correct air leaks in endotracheal, tracheostomy cuff, ventilator system • Check all tubing connections • Inflate cuff as needed for leaks • Reevaluate ventilator to make sure patient is receiving prescribed tidal volume
Low inspiratory pressure	• Air leaks causing volume loss • Tidal volume too low for the patient (often so because of a tendency to prescribe low tidal volumes)	• Assess, correct air leaks in endotracheal, tracheostomy cuff, ventilator system • Recheck ventilator to make sure prescribed tidal volume is delivered
Apnea	• True apnea, unstable ventilatory drive because of medications depressing central nervous system	• Ventilate manually as needed • May need to switch to mode that provides more ventilation support

Adapted from references 15 and 25

apnea". Apnea can only be assessed after stimulation of the respiratory centers. On the basis of animal experiments and clinical observations, a target $PaCO_2$ of 60 mm Hg has been proposed as a level at which the respiratory centers are maximally stimulated. However, it has been assumed that the respiratory centers are reset higher due to malfunction from brainstem injury. With oxygen administration, $PaCO_2$ increases. The increase in $PaCO_2$ is biphasic, with a steep increase in the first minutes due to equilibration of arterial carbon dioxide with mixed central

> **BY THE WAY**
>
> - Respiratory rhythm does not closely localize to specific regions
> - No single ventilatory parameter can be judged in isolation
> - Central hyperventilation is common and muted best with opioids
> - Adjust ventilator settings using blood gas values and patient comfort
> - Failure to trigger the ventilator is more often attributable to the machine setting than the patient effort

> **BREATHING BY THE NUMBERS**
>
> - ~ 50% decrease in volume or pressures requires assisted ventilation
> - ~ 30% change in vital capacity with position change indicates poor mechanics
> - ~ 30% of pulmonary shunting requires mechanical ventilation
> - ~ 25% of acutely ill ventilated neurologic patients require tracheostomy
> - ~ 20% of patients with acute brain injury have Cheyne-Stokes breathing

venous carbon dioxide. In the tracheobronchial phase of the apnea test, oxygen flow ensures uptake of oxygen in pulmonary capillaries; however, carbon dioxide exhalation does not take place and, therefore, there is a rapid rise of $PaCO_2$ due to metabolic production of carbon dioxide. Increase in $PaCO_2$ results in a decrease in CSF pH, which is sensed by the medullary respiratory centers, and when function is present results in a respiratory drive. Only a rapid increase in $PaCO_2$ to 60 mm Hg or 20 mm Hg above normal baseline values maximally stimulates these centers, also because CSF is unable to buffer acidosis with blood bicarbonate owing to its slower diffusion than carbon dioxide.

PUTTING IT ALL TOGETHER

- The pneumotaxic center regulates tidal volume and respiratory rate
- Ventilation is stimulated after PO_2 is less than 60 mm Hg
- Inability to cough up secretions, tachypnea, hemodynamic instability, and abnormal arterial blood gas with abnormal $PaCO_2$ or PaO_2 are all indications for intubation and mechanical ventilation
- Noninvasive mechanical ventilation is not often helpful in acute neurologic disease but may be tried
- Ventilator dyssynchrony is often noticed by high pressures and not much moving volume
- Weaning in patients with acute neurologic disease remains poorly standardized

References

1. Angus DC. When should a mechanically ventilated patient undergo tracheostomy? *JAMA* 2013;309:2163–2164.
2. Blum AS, Inves JR, Goldberger AL, et al. Oxygen desaturations triggered by partial seizures: implications of cardiopulmonary instability in epilepsy. *Epilepsia* 2000;41:536–541.
3. Blum AS. Respiratory physiology of seizures. *J Clin Neurophysiol* 2009;26:309–315.
4. Corfield DR, Fink JR, Ramsay SC, et al. Evidence for limbic system activation during CO_2 stimulated breathing in man. *J Physiol* 1995;488:77–84.
5. Corfield DR, Murphy K, Guz A. Does the motor cortical control of the diaphragm "bypass" the brainstem respiratory centres in men? *Respir Physiol* 1998;114:109–117.
6. Coulter DL. Partial seizures with apnea and bradycardia. *Arch Neurol* 1984;41:173–174.
7. Evans KC, Shea SA, Saykin AJ. Functional MRI localization of central nervous system regions associated with volitional inspirations in humans. *J Physiol* 1999;520:383–392.
8. Feldman Jl, Mitchell GS, Nattie EE. Breathing: rhythmicity, plasticity, chemosensitivity. *Annu Rev Neurosci* 2003;26:239–266.
9. Feldman JL. Looking forward to breathing.*Prog Brain Res* 2011;188:213–218.
10. Gozal D, Hathout GM, Kirlew KAT, et al. Localization of putative neural respiratory regions in the human by functional magnetic resonance imaging. *J Appl Physiol* 1994;76:2076–2083.
11. Hind CR. Neurogenic respiratory failure.*Handb Clin Neurol.* 2013;110:295–302.
12. Hess D. Noninvasive ventilation in neuromuscular disease: equipment and application. *Respiratory Care* 2006;51:896–911
13. Horn EM, Waldrop TG. Suprapontine control of respiration. *Respir Physiol* 1998;114:201–211.
14. Howard RS, Wiles CM, Hirsh NP, et al. Respiratory involvement in multiple sclerosis. *Brain* 1992;115:479–494.
15. Huang YT, Singh J. Basic modes of mechanical ventilation. In: Peters J, Papadakos B, eds. *Mechanical Ventilation: Clinical Applications and Pathophysiology*. Philadelphia, PA: Saunders, 2008. 247–268.
16. Jackson JH. On asphyxia in slight epileptic paroxysms. *Lancet* 1899;153:79–80.
17. James MR, Marshall H, Carew-McColl M. Pulse oximetry during apparent tonic-clonic seizures. *Lancet* 1991;337:394–395.
18. MacIntyre NR, Branson RD. *Mechanical Ventilation* 2nd ed. Philadelphia (PA), Elsevier, 2009.
19. Mehta S, Hill N. Noninvasive ventilation. *Am J Respir Crit Care Med* 2001;163:540–577.
20. Nelson DA, Ray CD. Respiratory arrest from seizure discharges in limbic system. Report of cases. *Arch Neurol* 1968;19:199–207.
21. Neubauer JA, Sunderram J. Oxygen-sensing neurons in the central nervous system. *J Appl Physiol* 2004;96:367–374.
22. Putnam RW, Filosa JA, Ritucci NA. Cellular mechanisms involved in CO_2 and acid signaling in chemosensitive neurons. *Am J Physiol* 2004;287:C1493–C1526.
23. Struth EA, Stucke AG, Brades IF, Zuperku EJ. Anesthetic effects on synaptic transmissions and gain control in respiratory control. *Respir Physiol Neurobiol* 2008;164:151–159.
24. Teppema LJ, Baby S. Anesthetics and control of breathing. *Respir Physiol Neurobiol* 2011;177:80–92.
25. Tobin MJ. *Principles and Practice of Mechanical Ventilation* 2nd ed. New York (NY), McGraw-Hill, 2006.
26. Tobin MJ. Extubation and the myth of "minimal ventilator settings." *Am J Respir Crit Care Med* 2012;185:349–350

6

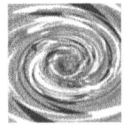

Neurology of Blood Pressure

The observation of a close link between acute brain injury and changes in blood pressure was one of the first fundamental discoveries in this field. Acute hypertension is a frequent accompanying clinical sign in any acute brain injury and is best known as the dire cerebral vasopressor response to increased intracranial pressure. It is also commonly interpreted as a nature's way to improve cerebral blood flow and for many decades there has been a concern treatment would do harm.[29]

Hypotension is far less common after acute brain injury and points to an associated medical or surgical problem (e.g. sepsis in fulminant meningitis, blood loss in polytrauma). Marked dehydration or sepsis are complication after acute brain injury and may result in rapidly refractory hypotension. Acute hypotension in catastrophic brain injury often indicates brain death.

Cerebral blood flow is generally held constant through a mechanism of autoregulation that allows adjustment of vascular diameter when blood pressure changes, but this regulatory response may not be adequate in acute brain injury.

So where do we like blood pressure levels to be at? The definition of "high" and "low" blood pressure depends on the type of brain injury. For example, in acute ischemic stroke there must be a balance between adequate perfusion of the penumbra and the risk of hemorrhage with breakthrough high blood pressures. Therefore, to appropriately manage blood pressure in any patient with an acute neurologic condition requires understanding of the physiology of cerebral perfusion pressure but also pharmacologic effects of vasopressors or antihypertensive drugs on the cerebral vasculature.[3,8]

There are imperative questions to answer: What makes the blood pressure go up and what makes it go down after acute brain injury? What are the target blood pressure values? What determines the choice of antihypertensive drugs? What do vasopressors do to the brain vasculature? In this chapter, we discuss the principles of blood pressure management, its effects on cerebral perfusion, and specific management in certain disorders.

Principles

Blood pressure and cardiac function are influenced by the sympathetic and parasympathetic systems. Variability may increase with age due to changed cardiac function and changes in arterial compliance.

BLOOD PRESSURE AND THE BRAIN

Some basic information first. Transmission through sympathetic fibers takes place largely via norepinephrine, the most important neurotransmitter in sympathetic terminals. Epinephrine is released from adrenal cells in response to preganglionic input. The precursor of both norepinephrine and epinephrine is dopamine. Generally, the α-effect pertains to vasoconstriction (vasopressor effect) and the β-effect to increase in cardiac contractility (inotropic effect), and there are several major receptors.[28]

The α-1 receptor mediates sympathetic constriction of the vasculature. The α-2 receptor reduces smooth muscle contraction. The β-adrenergic receptors are divided into β-1 adrenergic receptors, which mediate stimulating sympathetic effects on heart rate, excitability, and contractility; β-2 receptors, which mediate smooth muscle relaxation; and β-3 adrenergic receptors, which trigger lipolysis in brown fat. The mechanism of action is shown in Table 6.1.

The most important receptors are therefore α-1 adrenergic receptors, located in the arteries; the α-1 and β-1 adrenergic receptors, in the heart; and the α-2 and β-2 adrenergic receptors, in the veins.

How does the sympathetic nervous system regulate the vasomotor tone? There are vasomotor centers in the brainstem that receive input from the glossopharyngeal nerve and vagus nerve through carotid baroreceptors.[28] The sympathoexcitatory neurons of the rostral ventrolateral medulla maintain a vascular tone. These neurons also send fibers to the intermediolateral cell column in the spinal cord, connecting to sympathetic ganglions and arteries.

Table 6.1 **Mechanisms of Action**

α-1	α-2	β-1	β-2
Vasoconstriction	Sphincter contraction (GI)	Increased cardiac output (contraction and heart rate)	Arterial dilation (muscle)
Bronchoconstriction			Bronchodilation
Sphincter contraction (U)	Platelet aggregation		Sphincter relaxation

U: urosphincters; GI: Gastrointestinal

More recently it has become clear that there are also caudal medulla oblongata pressure areas.

More specifically, the sympathetic system controls three major contributors to the blood pressure: heart rate, heart contractility through stroke volume, and peripheral vasoconstriction that makes up the total peripheral resistance. The baroreceptors are located in the aorta, carotid sinus, and the heart—with changes in arterial pressure, they give afferent input into the autonomic centers of the brain that result in reflex changes in both sympathetic and parasympathetic activity. When the arterial pressure is decreased, the baroreceptors sense a decrease in stretch that then results in a decrease in baroreceptor input to the nucleus tractus solitarius. This decrease in input increases the sympathetic activity and inhibition of the parasympathetic activity[4,30] (Figure 6.1).

Now knowing what part of the brain is involved with blood pressure control, we need to know how blood pressure affects the cerebral circulation. It has been known for decades that manipulating blood pressure leads to changes in pial vasomotor responses. Information about cerebral autoregulation of the vascular tone came with the classic experiment by Lassen, who used controlled hypotension and simultaneously measured cerebral blood flow at the same time. It was found that there is a certain range of pressures with similar cerebral blood flow, suggesting an autoregulation mechanism separated by lower and upper blood pressure limits.[35]

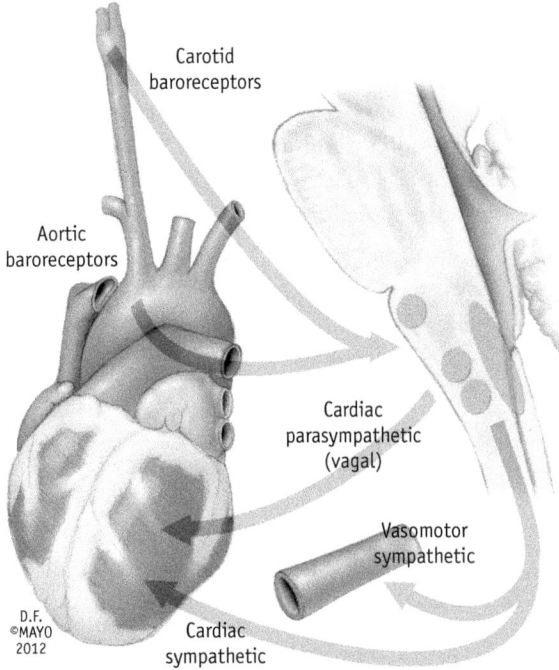

Figure 6.1 Parasympathetic and sympathetic input to heart and vessels.

This autoregulatory system is depicted in Figure 6.2. When the cerebral perfusion pressure falls below 50 mm Hg, the cerebral blood flow falls more or less linearly and may reach a flow rate that will be insufficient.[27] Hypoperfusion may lead to neuronal breakdown and spreading depression that may lead to cell death with prolonged depolarization (Chapter 1).[11] At the other end of the spectrum, when the cerebral perfusion pressure exceeds 150 mm Hg there is no further possibility for arterial vasoconstriction, by which point arteries have come under significant pressure. Above this upper limit of autoregulation, the resistance arteries are unable to maintain the vasoconstriction and a so-called sausage stringing, with dilated segments and local areas of constriction, is observed that eventually will lead to more dilatation of the arterial bed and passive increase of the cerebral blood flow.[19] These arteries may become leaky, and vasogenic edema may occur.

Long-standing hypertension could shift this curve to the right, changing these limits. The shift to higher values in patients with long-standing hypertension may be a result of a protective effect, but is also problematic when blood pressure is reduced, resulting in ischemia at comparatively high blood pressures.

Autoregulation is most likely controlled by smooth muscle in the resistance arteries that respond to changes in perfusion pressure; this smooth muscle contracts when that pressure increases and relaxes when there is hypotension. There are other mechanisms that include the release of vasoactive substances such as carbon dioxide, hydrogen ions, oxygen, adenosine, potassium, and calcium, but this response is likely slow and not as quick as a myogenic response.

It has been traditionally known that cerebral blood flow is coupled to neurometabolism; increase in neuron activity results in an increase in glucose utilization that also results in increased cerebral blood flow. Markedly decreased cerebral blood flow could potentially lead to ischemia, but even if the blood pressure would fall to the lower limit of autoregulation, the brain could compensate by increasing

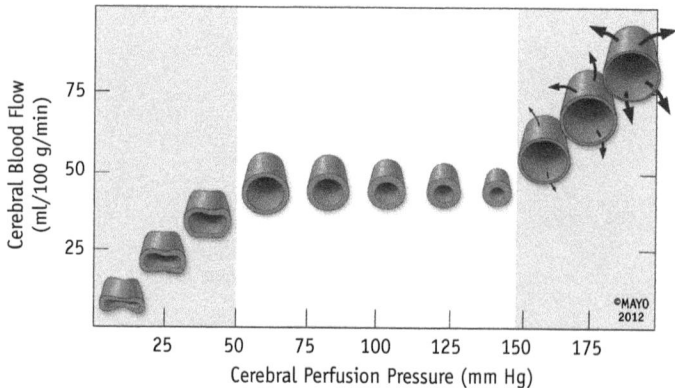

Figure 6.2 Autoregulation zone and changes in blood vessel diameter in relation to blood pressure.

oxygen extraction from perfusing blood. As a reference, normally constant cerebral blood flow is 50 mL/100 g/min and there is little change between cerebral perfusion pressures of 60 to 100 mm Hg. Cerebral blood flow is correlated to changes in neuronal function. At first protein synthesis is inhibited, usually with cerebral blood flow of 50 mL/100 g/min. When the flow rates are <35 mL/100 g/min, glucose utilization declines, even more at 25 mL/100 g/min.[22] At this point, there is anaerobic glycolysis with acidosis and lactate accumulation. Anoxic depolarization with changes in potassium and calcium is usually seen with cerebral blood flow at <15 mL/100 g/min.

Autoregulation is also regulated by $PaCO_2$ and PaO_2.[30] In general, an increase in CO_2 of 1 mm Hg changes the cerebral blood flow by only 5%. Oxygen fluctuations do not affect cerebral blood flow, but when PaO_2 is below 50 mm Hg, the cerebral blood flow will increase significantly.

The relationship between intracranial pressure and blood pressure is reasonably well understood.[7] We all know from seeing patients suddenly deteriorating from a new hemorrhage that blood pressure suddenly increases when the intracranial pressure suddenly rises. In more scientific terms, it is now understood as a state of sympathoactivation secondary to medullary hypoxia mediated by depolarization of rostral ventrolateral medulla neurons.[4]

When intracranial pressure is increased, further increasing the blood pressure will increase the brain elastance and further increase cerebral blood flow.[8] When arterial blood pressure is decreased in the setting of increased intracranial pressure, the brain elastance decreases, but cerebral blood flow also decreases, potentially causing ischemic changes.[22]

BLOOD PRESSURE AND DRUGS THAT MANIPULATE IT

In acutely ill brain-injured patients, blood pressure can swing in both directions—vasopressor and antihypertensive drugs are both commonly used.[26,34] Acute antihypertensive therapy is different from long-term antihypertensive therapy and requires interventions with different drugs. Most commonly used drugs in the emergency department or intensive care units are β-blockers and calcium channel blockers. Loop diuretics are also used, typically for conditions with fluid overload. Thiazide-type diuretics are more commonly used for long-term control of hypertension.[33]

β-blockers (also known as β-adrenergic blocking agents or β-antagonists) reduce heart rate and cardiac output, inhibit renin release, reduce venous return and plasma volume, reduce peripheral vascular resistance, and reset baroreceptor levels; all of these effects create antihypertensive action.[13] The drugs most commonly used are labetalol (additional α-1 adrenergic blocking activity and direct vasodilatory activity due to β-2 agonism); metoprolol, with a relative β-1 selectivity; or atenolol, with similar β-1 selectivity as metoprolol. The β-1 selective agents are safer than nonselective agents because β-blockers can worsen bronchospasm in patients with chronic obstructive pulmonary disease. β-blockers are also well known to reduce perioperative myocardial ischemia and provide protection against perioperative cardiovascular complications. This applies most often to patients undergoing vascular surgery who have a documented ischemic heart disease or other multiple risk factors.

β-blockers may worsen glucose intolerance and also mask the symptoms of hypoglycemia. Sudden discontinuation of β-blockers to allow for permissive hypertension after admission of ischemic stroke may cause rebound tachycardia with demand ischemia. β-blockers combined with diltiazem or verapamil may depress its effect on the sinoatrial and atrial ventricular nodes, and cause negative inotropy.

Angiotensin receptor blockers are often considered in patients with diabetic nephropathy, chronic heart failure, or congestive heart failure after myocardial infarction.[13,14,18,20,37] The drugs are most effective in combination with thiazide diuretics or calcium channel blockers. The commonly used drug is losartan. The drug is frequently made in three drug combinations, adding it with amlodipine or HCTZ.

Calcium channel blockers inhibit calcium flux and cause relaxation of vascular smooth muscle, resulting in vasodilatation and reduction of blood pressure. Calcium channel blockers reduce contractility of cardiac muscle and also slow the sinus pacemaker and atrioventricular conduction.[12] Calcium channel blockers are commonly used in neurologic settings. Examples are nifedipine, diltiazem, verapamil, and nimodipine. Calcium channel blockers are not prescribed for patients at high risk for cardiac failure due to abnormal left ventricular function. The drug that is frequently used long term is amlodipine. Diltiazem is often used to control ventricular rhythm, but this is contraindicated in patients with acute myocardial infarction and pulmonary congestion.

Another available drug in the acute setting is hydralazine, a powerful vasodilator that works via increase of cyclic guanosine monophosphate. It causes an increase in heart rate, making it a useful drug in patients with acute brain injury and bradycardia.

The commonly used drug sodium nitroprusside potently dilates cerebral arteries and veins and has been associated with increased intracranial pressure. There is also significant concern regarding toxicity of cyanide and thiocyanate, and therefore its use as an antihypertensive drug is discouraged.

A central sympatholytic drug is clonidine, but is rarely used for treatment of acute hypertension. Clonidine, however, is very effective in paroxysmal sympathetic hyperactivity syndrome associated with hypertensive surges. Clonidine decreases cardiac output by approximately 20% without any effect on peripheral resistance.[6,16] The central sympatholytic effect is produced via activation of the α-adrenergic receptor in the rostral ventral lateral medulla, and that mechanism results in decreased heart rate, cardiac output, and total peripheral resistance. It also has been known to activate the α-2 receptors in vascular smooth muscle and therefore may cause transient vasoconstriction and blood pressure elevation if the drug is administered acutely. The dose typically used in patients with hypertensive surges is 0.2 to 1.2 mg/day and has a maximal effect of 1 to 4 hours with a half-life of 6 to 16 hours.

With all these drugs available in the acute setting, either labetalol, esmolol, nicardipine, or hydralazine can be used, and the rule of 10 applies; 10 mg IV of each of these drugs is a good starting dose and will show if the drug is effective and whether repeated doses are needed.

Hypotension in acute brain injury is most commonly due to dehydration as a result of large amount of unmeasurable fluid loss (fever, nutrition associated diarrhea, mechanical ventilation). Fluid resuscitation is the first approach, but hypotension may require administration of vasoactive drugs. Vasoactive drugs often have both vasopressor and inotropic actions and thus not only raise blood pressure but also raise cardiac output. Clinically, hypotension presents itself with, oliguria, delayed capillary refill, and cooling of the skin. In addition there is elevated serum lactate and often evidence of decreased mixed venous oxyhemoglobin saturation. The mixed venous oxyhemoglobin saturation is a reflection of the balance between oxygen delivery and consumption, and, therefore, decreased oxyhemoglobin saturation is indicative of poor organ perfusion. Another measure of adequate resuscitation is measurement of central venous pressure.

The major vasoactive agents are shown in Table 6.2,[17] and the relative contribution of α- and β-effects is shown in Figure 6.3. The goal is to maintain mean arterial blood pressure above 60 mm Hg. Vasopressors are usually phenylephrine and norepinephrine. Phenylephrine is a selective α-1 adrenergic receptor agonist and can augment blood pressure. The drug does not cause tachydysrhythmias and is usually started at 50 mcg/min. Norepinephrine is a potent α-2 adrenergic receptor agonist but also a β-1 receptor agonist, and thus results in tachycardia; therefore, it can be used in patients with bradycardia. However, tachydysrhythmia can occur with doses up to 30 mcg/min. Norepinephrine is a potent vasoconstrictor and is considered a first-line vasopressor in patients with shock. When norepinephrine is compared with dopamine, mortality is lower with norepinephrine in patients with cardiogenic shock.[24] It should be noted that most vasopressive agents can result in tachycardia. This may lead to demand ischemia in patients who have prior coronary artery disease. In patients who have a troponin increase or electrographic changes, vasopressors can be combined with dobutamine as an additional inotropic agent.

Dopamine has pharmacologic effects that are dose dependent. At lower doses the β-1 adrenergic effects increase cardiac contractility and heart rate, but at higher doses (above 10 mcg/kg/min) α-effects are more predominant, resulting in arterial vasoconstriction and increase in blood pressure. Dopamine has the disadvantage that more arrhythmic events are seen than in patients treated with norepinephrine.[9]

Table 6.2 **Commonly Used Vasoactive Agents**

| | | Cardiac | | Peripheral Vasculature | |
	Dose	Rate	Contractility	Vasoconstriction	Vasodilation
Norepinephrine	2–40 µg/min	+	++	++++	0
Dopamine	1–4 µg/kg/min	+	+	0	+
	4–20 µg/kg/min	++	++/+++	++/+++	0
Epinephrine	1–20 µg/min	++++	++++	++++	+++
Phenylephrine	20–200 µg/min	0	0	+++	0
Vasopressin	0.01–0.03 U/min	0	0	++++	0
Dobutamine	2–20 µg/kg/min	++	+++/++++	0	++
Milrinone	0.375–0.75 µg/kg/min	+	+++	0	++

Adapted from reference 17.

Phenylephrine also increases blood pressure through vasoconstriction and usually a single intravenous dose of 100-200 mcg is successful in increasing blood pressure. Phenylephrine, however, is a good option when tachyarrhythmias occur with other vasopressors. Phenylephrine is the preferred drug in spinal shock and in patients who have systemic vasodilatation.

A separate issue is whether vasopressors can affect the brain vasculature.[23,31,32,36,38] Again, phenylephrine is an α-1 adrenergic agonist; norepinephrine acts as both α- and β-adrenergic receptors and causes vasoconstriction. Dopamine typically stimulates dopaminergic and β-adrenergic receptors at low and moderate doses and α-adrenergic receptors at higher doses. However the intracerebral vessels have low α-receptor densities. Phenylephrine may lead to decreased

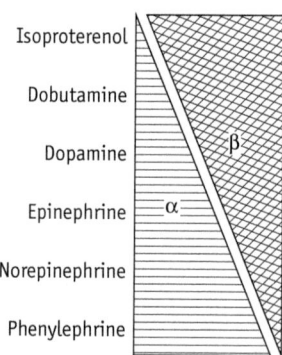

Figure 6.3 α and β effect of vasopressors and inotropes. (Adapted from reference 17.)

cerebral oxygenation; but a direct action of phenylephrine or epinephrine on cerebral resistance vessels is not present also because these vasoactive drugs do not cross the blood-brain barrier.[26]

Vasopressin has been considered an important drug, particularly when added to norepinephrine, and has been quite successful in resuscitation of patients with septic shock, mainly to reduce the dose of norepinephrine.

Vasopressin has the advantage of having (1) no evidence of cerebral vasoconstriction, (2) no impact on cardiac output, (3) no reflexive increase in vagal tone, and (4) fewer cardiac arrhythmias associated with vasopressors and improved coronary flow in the absence of vasopressors, and long term it may even reverse adrenergic receptor down-regulation (increase water reabsorption due to increasing permeability of the collecting ducts) via constriction of vascular smooth muscle.

The best-known inotropic agent is dobutamine. This is typically used in patients with cardiogenic shock. It is much less often used in patients who are hypotensive as the response is unpredictable because of lower vasopressor effects. Dobutamine also causes tachyarrhythmia and can provoke myocardial ischemia. Dobutamine can be used when echocardiogram shows markedly reduced ejection fraction or for patients who are in septic shock.[2]

A new interesting drug is milrinone, which has significant inotropic effects. It is typically used in cardiogenic shock and in patients who need treatment for acute cardiac failure. Milrinone is a potent pulmonary vasodilator and has the potential to worsen hypotension. Some centers have used milrinone to increase cerebral perfusion pressure. Milrinone has a 2- to 4-hour half-life but may cause thrombocytopenia. It is also a good alternative if there is a long-term need for β-agonists.

In Practice

Treatment of hypertension and hypotension is commonly needed in acutely ill neurologic patients, although not at the level of intensity required in medically ill patients.

ACUTE HYPERTENSION MANAGEMENT

The discussion of unacceptable hypertension requires definitions of "unacceptable" and "hypertension." "Unacceptable" describes any blood pressure that may cause worsening from rehemorrhage, cerebral edema, ventricular strain, or cardiac arrhythmias. "Hypertension" is understood as a blood pressure that is too high under the circumstances. Here are some recommendation from major medical societies. Patients who are candidates for thrombolysis need to have their hypertension controlled by reducing the systolic blood pressure below 185 mm Hg and the diastolic blood pressure below 110 mm Hg. Patients with intracerebral hemorrhage should be treated to achieve moderate blood pressure reduction (systolic blood pressure <180–160 mm Hg, mean arterial pressure <130–110 mm Hg). The recent long awaited ATACH 2 study found little, if any, benefit in rapid lowering of blood pressure to 140 mm Hg systolic range and maintaining it for a week.[1] In aneurysmal subarachnoid hemorrhage, many practitioners prefer to treat hypertension with the goal of maintaining the systolic blood pressure below 160–180 mm Hg before the aneurysm is secured. But when the literature is scrutinized for guidance, it reveals a bedeviling number of blood pressure targets.

Extreme hypertension is avoided for many reasons, and antihypertensives may be used intravenously to that end. Management of hypertension using IV agents is a common reason to transfer patients to an ICU or keep them in the ICU. Labetalol is preferred for treatment of acute hypertension. The cardiac output is maintained with blockers of both α and β receptors and therefore not changed with labetalol. Bradycardia might be a side effect of labetalol, but the drug can be administered in 20- to 40-mg IV boluses. Some have used a continuous infusion of 0.5 mg/min to control hypertension. An alternative drug is esmolol, a selective antagonist of β-1 adrenergic receptors. Esmolol may produce more significant bradyarrhythmias or hypotension and the effect lasts only 10 minutes. An infusion of 25 mcg/kg/min increasing to 300 mcg/kg/min can be used to control hypertension. The third drug is nicardipine, a calcium channel blocker that produces peripheral arterial vasodilatation, but again it does not cause cardiac arrhythmias and thus is an ideal drug for blood pressure reduction without having the risk of bradydysrhythmias. Nicardipine can be successful with an intravenous dose of 5 mg/h to 15 mg/h and may dampen acute blood pressure variability so commonly seen with other IV antihypertensives. Blood pressure management with IV nicardipine is currently investigated in cerebral hemorrhage.

In any acute devastating neurologic disorder, there is an increase in sympathetic activity. Hypertension, tachyarrhythmias, hypothermia, and hyperhidrosis are clinical presentations. This sympathetic hyperactivity can occur with massive lesions in the cortex, diencephalon, and brainstem but also with lesions in the spinal cord. Spinal cord injury above the T-5 level can lead to a significant activity of the sympathoexcitatory reflexes and lead to autonomic dysreflexia, which is noted by extreme hypertension and sudden cardiac arrhythmias.

These spells, also known as sympathetic storm, are best treated with propranolol, clonidine, dexmedetomidine (another central α-2 receptor agonist), bromocriptine (a dopamine D2-receptor agonist), baclofen (a $GABA_B$ receptor agonist), benzodiazepines ($GABA_A$ receptor agonist), but most successfully with high doses of gabapentin (which binds GABA receptors and voltage-gated calcium channels in the dorsal horn of the spinal cord).

ACUTE HYPOTENSION MANAGEMENT

Traditional teaching explains acute hypotension as caused by cardiogenic, vasodilatory (distributory), or hypovolemic shock. In acute neurologic conditions one can see these causes in CNS infections with septicemia, profound blood loss in traumatic head injury with fractures or abdominal trauma, and cardiac dysfunction from neurogenic stress cardiomyopathy. Cardiogenic shock is best first treated with dobutamine and dopamine (in combination) to improve inotropy (often at a dose of 7.5 µg/kg/min each). Norepinephrine is needed if this does not result in blood pressure stabilization (systolic blood pressure < 70 mm Hg). In vasodilatory shock, epinephrine or norepinephrine is used and frequently combined with vasopressin.

Hypotension may be due to dehydration. Dehydration may be diagonised by oliguria (0.5 ml/kg/hour) or increase in blood urea nitrogen (BUN)/creatinine ratio (more that 20). Treatment is saline resuscitation often upto 5 liters initially (minimum 30 ml/kg).[10] The usual target is a mean arterial pressure of 65 mm Hg. A serum lactic acid can be used as guidance and a level > 4 mmol/L indicates tissue hypoperfusion and calls for aggressive hemodynamic support.

Norepinephrine is supplemented with low-dose vasopressin (0.03 units per minute) if the blood pressure target is not achieved. Phenylephrine is not a good choice in septic shock because it can reduce cardiac output and with sepsis patients may already have myocardial dysfunction. Patients with septic shock not quickly responding to these measures may be treated with corticosteroids (hydrocortisone 50 mg intravenously every 6 hours). Intravenous hydrocortisone is only needed if blood pressure remains unstable.[10] In patients with vasodilatory shock, aggressive fluid resuscitation (quick administration of 1–2 liter of crystalloids or transfusion of red blood cells) is first used. Early use of albumin in severe sepsis can be considered as a resuscitative measure. Because sodium and water overload may lead to interstitial edema and organ dysfunction and continuous fluid resuscitation should be avoided once rehydration is achieved.[25]

Hypotension is often a clear defining sign of brain death after a catastrophic neurologic injury. Loss of sympathetic tone and vasodilation contribute to blood pressure instability. Hemodynamic instability, however, is more likely a result of reduced afterload than poor cardiac contractility. The approach includes fluid resuscitation, administration of packed red cells if the hemoglobin level is less than 9 and the hematocrit is less than 30%, correction of any hypothermia, and use of vasopressors. If the patient becomes an organ donor some protocols include norepinephrine; others include dopamine or dobutamine, alone or in combination with vasopressin.[9]

> **BY THE WAY**
>
> - Goals of adequate blood pressure in acute brain injury have not been defined
> - Control of systolic blood pressure to less than 160 mm Hg is safe in most patients with acute brain injury
> - Hypertensive surges needs control and may not be "compensatory" in acute brain injury
> - All patients with major acute blood pressure problems need central venous and arterial access
> - With hypotension the sequence is: volume correction with crystalloids, colloids, or volume expander such as albumen followed next by a β-agonist (dopamine) before adding an α-agonist (phenylephrine)

> **NEUROLOGY OF BLOOD PRESSURE BY THE NUMBERS**
>
> - ~ 95% of epinephrine is α-action
> - ~ 95% of dobutamine is β-action
> - ~ 80% of acute hypertension is controlled with β-blockers
> - ~ 50% increase in systemic blood pressure with 500-cc fluid bolus
> - ~ 10% increase in systemic blood pressure in Trendelenburg

Putting It All Together

- α-effects are vasoconstriction; β-effects are inotropic or cause vasodilation
- Dopamine and dobutamine are inotropic; phenylephrine and epinephrine are vasoconstrictive
- Hypotension is treated first with fluid resuscitation followed by norepinephrine
- Combining inotropes and vasopressors may avoid adverse effects of each drug at high doses
- Vasopressin is an ideal "catecholamine sparing agent" and should be considered if long-term management is anticipated

References

1. Anderson CS, Heeley E, Huang Y, et al. Rapid blood-pressure lowering in patients with acute intracerebral hemorrhage. *N Engl J Med* 2013;368:2355–2365.

2. Annane D, Vignon P, Renault A, et al. Norepinephrine plus dobutamine versus epinephrine alone for management of septic shock: a randomised trial. *Lancet* 2007;370:676–684.
3. Badruddin A, Taqi MA, Abraham MG, Dani D, Zaidat OO. Neurocritical care of a reperfused brain. *Curr Neurol Neurosci Rep* 2011;11:104–110.
4. Benarroch EE. The arterial baroreflex: functional organization and involvement in neurologic disease. *Neurology* 2008;71:1733–1738.
5. Berry C, Ley EJ, Bukur M, Malinoski D, Margulies DR, Mirocha J, Salim A. Redefining hypotension in traumatic brain injury. *Injury* 2012;43:1833–1837.
6. Cohn JN, McInnes GT, Shepherd AM. Direct-acting vasodilators. *J Clin Hypertension* 2011;13:690–692.
7. Czosnyka M, Brady K, Reinhard M, Smielewski P, Steiner LA. Monitoring of cerebrovascular autoregulation: facts, myths, and missing links. *Neurocrit Care* 2009;10:373–386.
8. Dagal A, Lam IS. Cerebral blood flow and the injured brain: how should we monitor and manipulate it? *Curr Opin Anaesthesiol* 2011;24:131–137.
9. De Backer D, Biston P, Devriendt J, et al. Comparison of dopamine and norepinephrine in the treatment of shock. *N Engl J Med* 2010;362:779–789.
10. Dellinger RP, Levy MM, Rhodes A, et al. Surviving sepsis campaign: international guidelines for management of severe sepsis and septic shock: 2012. *Crit Care Med*. 2013;41:580–637.
11. Dreier JP, Victorov IV, Petzold GC, et al. Electrochemical failure of the brain cortex is more deleterious when it is accompanied by low perfusion. *Stroke.* 2013;44:490–496.
12. Elliott WJ, Ram CVS. Calcium channel blockers. *J Clin Hypertension.* 2011;13:687–689.
13. Epstein M, Calhoun DA. Aldosterone blockers and potassium sparing diuretics. *J Clin Hypertens (Greenwich)* 2011;13:644–648.
14. Fisher NDL, Meagher EA. Renin inhibitors. *J Clin Hypertens* 2011;13:662–666.
15. Frishman WR, Saunders E. Beta-adrenergic blockers. *J Clin Hypertension* 2011;13:649–653.
16. Grimm RH, Flack JM. Alpha 1 adrenoreceptor antagonists. *J Clin Hypertension.* 2011;13:654–657.
17. Hollenberg SM. Vasoactive drugs in circulatory shock. *Am J Respir Crit Care Med* 2010;183:847–855.
18. Hollenberg SM, Parrillo JE. Acute heart failure and shock. In: Crawford MH, DeMarco J, Paulus WJ, eds. *Cardiology* 3rd ed. Philadelphia, Mosby, 2010.
19. Immink RV, van den Born BJ, van Montfrans GA, Koopmans RP, Karemaker JM, van Lieshout JJ. Impaired cerebral autoregulation in patients with malignant hypertension. *Circulation* 2004;11:2241–2245.
20. Izzo JL, Weir MR. Angiotensin-converting enzyme inhibitors. *J Clin Hypertension* 2011;13:667–675.
21. Koenig MA, Geocadin RG, de Grouchy M, et al. Safety of induced hypertension therapy in patients with acute ischemic stroke. *Neurocrit Care* 2006;4:3–7.
22. Markus HS. Cerebral perfusion and stroke. *J Neurol Neurosurg Psychiatry* 2004;75:353–361.
23. Meng L, Cannesson M, Alexander BS, et al. Effect of phenylephrine and ephedrine bolus treatment on cerebral oxygenation in anaesthetized patients. *Br J Anaesth* 2011;107:209–217.
24. Morelli A, Ertmer C, Rehberg S, et al. Phenylephrine versus norepinephrine for initial hemodynamic support of patients with septic shock: a randomized, controlled trial. *Crit Care* 2008;12:R143.
25. Myburgh JA, Mythen MG. Resuscitation fluids. *New Eng J Med* 2013;369:1243–1251.
26. Olesen J. The effect of intracarotid epinephrine, norepinephrine, and angiotensin on the regional cerebral blood flow in man. *Neurology* 1972;22:978–87.
27. Panerai RB. The critical closing pressure of the cerebral circulation. *Med Eng Phys* 2003;25:621–632.
28. Pilowsky PM, Goodchild AK. Baroreceptor reflex pathways and neurotransmitters: 10 years on. *J Hypertens* 2002;20:1675–1688.
29. Qureshi AI. The importance of acute hypertensive response in ICH. *Stroke.* 2013;44: S67–S69.

30. Rangel-Castilla L, Lara LR, Gopinath S, Swank PR, Valadka A, Robertson CJ. Cerebral hemodynamic effects of acute hyperoxia and hyperventilation after severe traumatic brain injury. *Neurotrauma* 2010;27:1853–1863.
31. Rordorf G, Cramer SC, Efird JT, Schwamm LH, Buonanno F, Koroshetz WJ. Pharmacological elevation of blood pressure in acute stroke. Clinical effects and safety. *Stroke* 1997; 28:2133–2138.
32. Rordorf G, Koroshetz WJ, Ezzeddine MA, Segal AZ, Buonanno FS. A pilot study of drug-induced hypertension for treatment of acute stroke. *Neurology* 2001;8;56:1210–1213.
33. Sica DA, Carter B, Cushman W, et al. Thiazide and loop diuretics. *J Clin Hypertension.* 2011;13:639–643.
34. Sookplung P, Siriussawakul A, Malakouti A, et al. Vasopressor use and effect on blood pressure after severe adult traumatic brain injury. *Neurocrit Care* 2011;15:46–54.
35. Strandgaard S, Paulson OB. Cerebral autoregulation. *Stroke* 1984;15:413–416.
36. Strandgaard S, Sigurdsson ST. Point: Counterpoint: Sympathetic activity does/does not influence cerebral blood flow. Counterpoint: Sympathetic nerve activity does not influence cerebral blood flow. *J Appl Physiol* 2008;105:1366–1367.
37. Taylor AA, Siragy H, Nesbitt SD. Angiotensin receptor blockers: pharmacology, efficacy and safety. *J Clin Hypertension.* 2011;13:677–686.
38. Van Lieshout JJ, Secher NH. Point: Counterpoint: Sympathetic activity does/does not influence cerebral blood flow. Point: Sympathetic activity does influence cerebral blood flow. *J Appl Physiol 2008*;105:1364–1366.
39. Vongpatanasin W, Kario K, Atlas SA, et al. Central sympatholytic drugs. *J Clin Hypertension.* 2011;13:658–661.
40. White H, Venkatesh B. Cerebral perfusion pressure in neurotrauma: a review. *Anesth Analg* 2008;107:979–988.
41. Zafar SN, Millham FH, Chang Y, et al. Presenting blood pressure in traumatic brain injury: a bimodal distribution of death. *J Trauma* 2011;71:1179–1184.

7

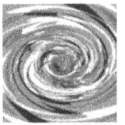

Neurology of Cardiac Function

The heartbeat is influenced by both sympathetic and parasympathetic nerve signals, and there is important interplay between these systems that have consequences for heart rate and contractility. These neuronal pathways are fundamentally the basis of the heart-brain connection.[29,30]

It is widely accepted that acute neurologic conditions often involve acute cardiac manifestations, and there is some understanding of its mechanism.[8,27] Acute neurologic injury may cause cardiac injury through a sympathetic overdrive originating from the anterior hypothalamus.[22] These stress-related cardiomyopathies are common in this situation and have presented themselves as acute left ventricular dysfunction.[35]

To try to understand how the heart becomes involved in neurologic disease, one must implicate excitation of the limbic system. When the limbic system—due to stress of any kind—is stimulated, the medullary autonomic center is activated, leading eventually to release of norepinephrine and epinephrine. The adrenal outflow of these catecholamines decreases the viability of cardiomyocytes through cyclic AMP and through immediate calcium overload and oxygen-derived free radicals.[5] Finding contraction band necrosis, neutrophil infiltration, and fibrosis has been considered a manifestation of a high concentration of calcium. The best correlation that has been found between cardiac dysfunction and elevated intracranial pressure (ICP) is in animal models showing that inducing an explosive rise in ICP will lead to a 1,000-fold increase in the level of epinephrine with greater areas of myocytolysis and necrosis, particularly when compared with gradual ICP increase.[32]

Physicians are understandably concerned by how acute brain injury may affect the heart. Not only is cardiac arrest associated with certain acute neurologic and neurosurgical conditions, but other cardiac manifestations undoubtedly catch the eye and may even need immediate intervention. So, we need to consider these questions: What is known about the heart-brain connection? What are the mechanisms at play? How serious are these transient cardiac arrhythmias and EKG changes? How should physicians respond to these manifestations?

This chapter will discuss the core fundamentals of cardiac injury from acute brain injury. We will also briefly touch on the effects of acute neuromuscular disorders.

Principles

The sinoatrial (SA) node—the major intrinsic cardiac pacemaker—receives a rich supply of both sympathetic and parasympathetic fibers. The atrioventricular (AV) node—the subsidiary pacemaker—also has both parasympathetic and sympathetic input, although not quite as extensive as in the SA node. Even more, the ventricles have a predominant sympathetic input with little parasympathetic contribution (Figure 7.1). Most of the nerves follow the pathway of the coronary arteries and end up in epicardial regions, mostly in the ventricles. The distribution of the nerve fibers is far more concentrated at the base than at the apex.

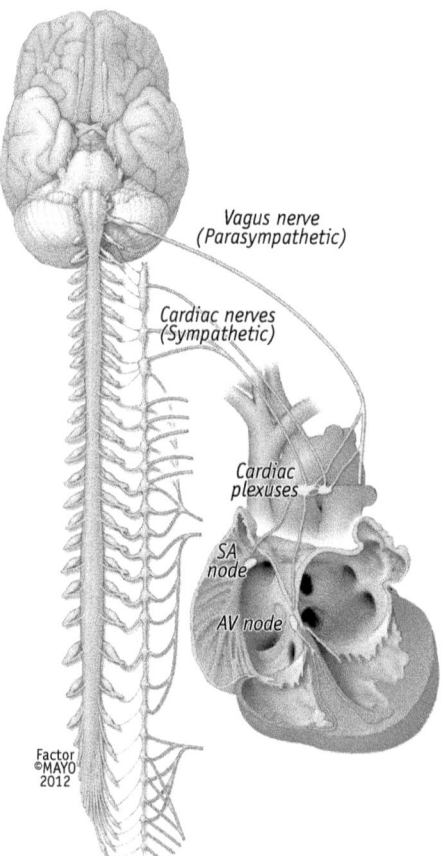

Figure 7.1 Sympathetic and parasympathetic input to cardiac conduction system.

Parasympathetic traffic increases the refractory period of the action potential. Sympathetic traffic does the opposite. Parasympathetic traffic (via the vagus nerve) makes conduction more difficult. Sympathetic traffic to the heart makes conduction easier.

Norepinephrine is the neurotransmitter of the sympathetic nerves and has positive inotropic (cardiac contraction) and chronotropic (increased heart rate) effects, but also causes coronary vasoconstriction. The sympathetic preganglion neurons that innervate the heart are usually derived from the T-1 to T-5 segments, and after projection to cervical and superior thoracic ganglia they provide axons to the cardiac plexus. Generally, the sympathetic fibers are spread throughout the heart and when norepinephrine attaches to the β-1 adrenergic receptor, the force and rate of contraction and the diastolic relaxation increases, eventually leading to better cardiac pump function. The heart rate increases as a result of both β-1 and β-2 receptor activation. The sympathetic overdrive results in increase in heart rate, increase in AV conduction, and increase in myocardial contractility. Right sympathetic traffic innervates the SA node and increases the heart rate, while left sympathetic traffic innervates the AV node and ventricle and increases the AV ventricular conduction.[3,9]

The normal resting condition favors vagal activity. Vagal stimulation releases acetylcholine, which binds to muscarinic receptors and causes a negative inotropic effect—this cholinergic effect decreases heart rate. Parasympathetic fibers are connected to the SA node, AV node, and atrial muscle via the vagus nerve. The right vagus branch maintain a beat-to-beat control of the heart rate; the left vagus branch controls AV conduction and myocardial excitability. Parasympathetic nerves decrease the heart rate via the SA node and decrease the action potential conduction velocity via the AV node. The force of the atrial muscle contraction also is decreased, which could lead to decreased cardiac pumping.

When the sympathetic system is charged, increased catecholamines may also lead to an increase in peripheral vascular resistance. The left ventricle has marked difficulties in overcoming this resistance, which would then lead to increased ventricular wall stress, in turn leading to electrical instability, resulting in ventricular tachyarrhythmias. In addition, a large increase in norepinephrine opens calcium channels and results in calcium influx and potassium efflux. Again, high levels of calcium could explain this hypercontracted state that eventually will lead to necrosis.

Under these circumstances cardiac muscle may start to show interstitial infiltration by polymorphonuclear leukocytes and macrophages and myocardial fibers may become separated. This myofibrillar degeneration is reminiscent of pheochromocytoma. Norepinephrine infusion may produce a similar finding and sympathectomy may prevent it.[26] There may be particular higher risk of stress cardiomyopathy if the negative feedback loop (afferent baroreflex) fails and the catecholamine surge is uncontrolled. This may occur in infarcts in the dorsal medulla oblongata that may interrupt signals to the nucleus tractus

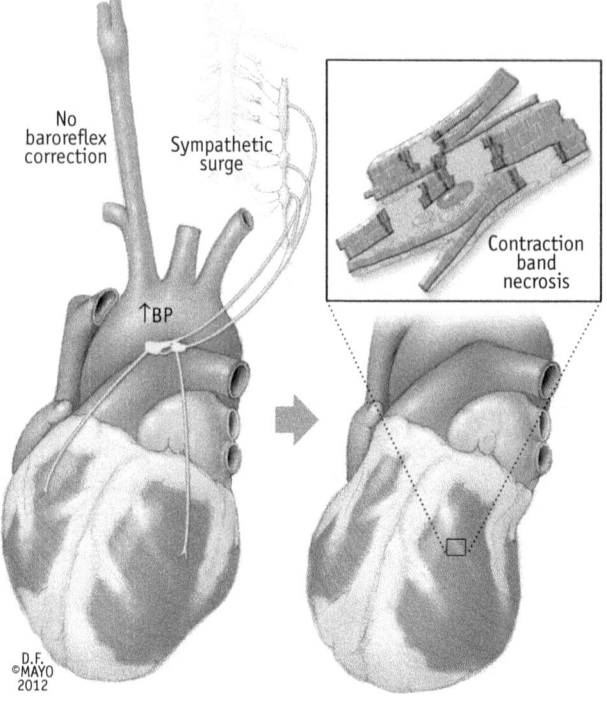

Figure 7.2 Mechanism of contraction band necrosis.

solitarius and in posterior reversible encephalopathy syndrome.[14] This possible mechanism is shown in Figure 7.2.

Knowing the major contribution of the autonomic system, it is important to review what stimulated part in the brain could specifically result in cardiac manifestations and what type. Again, increased sympathetic nerve output promotes arrhythmogenesis through variability in repolarization. Increased vagal tone induces bradycardia. Multiple areas in the brain can be implicated in cardiac arrhythmias. Structures that have received interest are the insular cortex, amygdala, caudate nucleus, periaqueductal gray; and specific areas in the medulla such as nucleus tractus solitarius (Figure 7.3).[10,25]

A relationship between insular cortex and cardiac arrhythmia is well known.[10] Experimental studies have found that damage to the nucleus tractus solitarius causes labile blood pressures and pathological changes in the pericardium that are characteristic of stress-induced myopathy.[25] Augmented sympathetic activity can create these abnormalities. Prior suggestions that multivessel coronary artery spasm may be causing these changes have been largely discounted.[34,37] This is also because none of the abnormalities follow the territory of coronary arteries, and are typically scattered and diffuse. Normal microvascular perfusion also

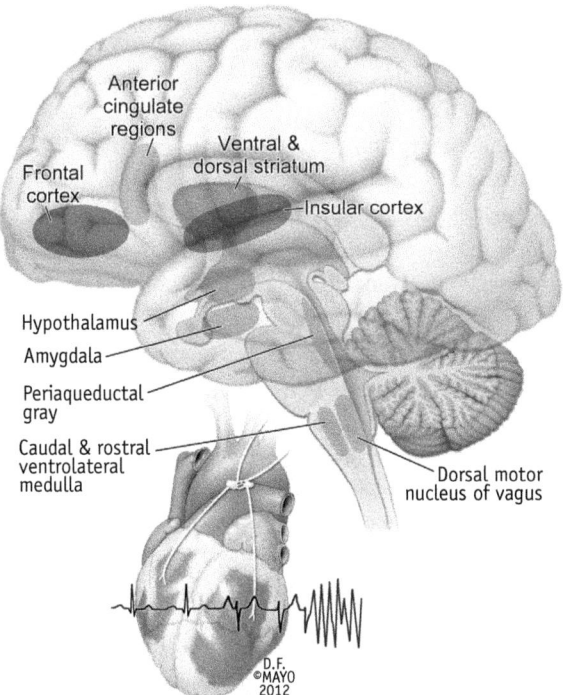

Figure 7.3 Brain areas implicated in cardiac arrhythmias.

argues against microvascular dysfunction, and in published reports perfusion in myocardium has not changed.[8,39]

There is also a suggestion that a hypothalamic connection might exist and a sympathetic activation could lead to perivascular hemorrhages and edema in myocardium.[26] Studies have found that peak values of CKMB and troponin T do correlate with peak values of neuroadrenaline and adrenaline, and there is also suggestion that the heart might be more sensitive to sympathetic stimulation in these conditions.[21,22] Microscopically myocardial contraction band necrosis or myocytolysis or myofibrillary degeneration can be seen as hypercontracted sarcomeres, dense eosinophilic transfers, bands, and an early interstitial mononuclear inflammatory response. Contraction band necrosis can be completely blocked by cardiac sympathectomy but is still present after a vagotomy and proves that intact vagal supply to the heart has no role. Contraction band necrosis also occurs after bilateral adrenalectomy, suggesting that the mediator of neurogenic cardiac injury is the local release of norepinephrine from myocardial sympathetic nerve terminals rather than circulating catecholamines.[24]

Experimental stimulation of the anterior hypothalamus may also result in ST segment depression on EKG. Clinically, however, this may become apparent via new EKG changes of the ST segment or T waves and a brief increase in serum troponin.

How the brain regulates (or better dysregulates) heart rate and rhythm remains partly elucidated. Arrhythmias are common after aneurysmal subarachnoid hemorrhage with no specific lesions, and any type of hemorrhagic stroke may trigger a new-onset atrial fibrillation. Most impressive is sudden death in epilepsy patients (SUDEP), due to ictal bradycardia and asystole.[23,29]

There is evidence of lateralization, and right insula and right anterior cingulate cortex may generate sympathetic overdrive as a result of stress or other emotions. The right-sided dominance for sympathetic effects on the heart has been consistently identified in experimental studies, but whether this exists in humans is not fully known.

Stimulation of rostral insular cortex results in a pressor effect, and caudal insular cortex irritability results in a depressor effect.[10] To add to the confusion, electrical stimulation of thalamus results in heart rate decrease and hypotension in rats, whereas the opposite occurs in humans.

When the sympathetic nerves or stellate ganglion are stimulated in experimental studies, the induced EKG repolarization reduces the fibrillation threshold, leading to ventricular fibrillation. Further evidence is that β-blockade can reverse these findings. Clonidine also reduces sympathetic drive and reduced the occurrences of ventricular tachycardia or ventricular fibrillation in experimental studies.

Cardiac physiology is also controlled by four other systems and feedback loops. First, as alluded to in Chapter 6, baroreceptor control modulates heart rate. The baroreceptors in the carotid sinus and aortic arch are stretched by an increase in mean arterial pressure, and there is a linear relation between increase in blood pressure and afferent discharge (the threshold is 60 mm Hg for the carotid and 90 mm Hg for the aortic arch). The baroreceptor afferent signal is integrated at the nucleus tractus solitarius and inhibits the sympathetic activation and excites the parasympathetic nerve.

Second, also in the carotid and aortic arch are chemoreceptors reacting to changes in pH, PO_2 or PCO_2, or temperature. Hypoxemia, hypercarbia, and acidosis will lead to increased heart rate, increased contractility, and cardiac output.

Third, mechanoreceptors are present in the heart. Atrial receptors usually respond to atrial distension with tachycardia (so-called Bainbridge reflex). The ventricular counterpart is the so-called Bezold–Jarisch reflex, which causes a depressor reflex (bradycardia, decreased contractility, and hypotension).

Fourth, the endocrine responses have become better characterized. Atrial natriuretic peptide is released in response to not only atrial β-receptor stimulation but also tachycardia. Atrial natriuretic peptide has a complex effect. It causes both arterial and venous dilatation and natriuresis with a reduction of aldosterone release through blockage of angiotensin II. Brain natriuretic peptide, synthesized in the ventricle, also produces natriuresis and is increased in cardiac failure and, thus, is a biomarker of ventricular failure. Infusion of brain natriuretic peptide has a positive hemodynamic effect in patients with cardiac failure.

Other neurohormones play a role, and vasopressin is also slightly increased in patients with cardiac failure, resulting in sodium retention and water retention causing hyponatremia. When measured, other hormones are increased; this includes neuropeptide Y and adrenomedullin. Their significance is not clearly understood.

In Practice

Some of the insights obtained by experimental studies can be translated to practice. All categories of acute heart failure may occur. Acute cardiac failure in acutely ill neurologic patients may have several causes and, thus, different approaches. Patients may have an acute decompensation of chronic heart failure, patients may have worsened from acute hypertension, patients may have developed a sudden decrease in ejection fraction with pulmonary edema, and some are rapidly going into cardiac shock. Ischemic heart disease from acute coronary syndromes may occur as a result of acute brain injury. Acute brain injury may also occur in a patient with a preexisting cardiac disorder. It calls to mind atrial fibrillation associated with ischemic stroke (if the patient is not anticoagulated) or cerebral hematoma (if the patient is anticoagulated).

Neurologists should recognize acute neurology-associated cardiac concerns. Here, we primarily discuss the recognition of common manifestations. Management is discussed in more detail in another volume of this series (*Providing Acute Care*).

NEUROGENIC CARDIAC FAILURE

Diagnosis of stress-induced cardiomyopathy is made on the basis of presence of arrhythmias (often tachycardia), EKG abnormalities (often QT prolongation and ST segment elevation), increased troponin levels (rapidly trending upward, though not as high as in a myocardial infarct), BNP (elevated), and chest X-ray (pulmonary edema often "flash" pulmonary edema). A transthoracic echocardiogram often shows marked reduction in ventricular function and regional wall motion abnormalities. If the regional wall motion abnormalities are beyond a single vascular territory and involve the apex (apical ballooning), a neurogenic stress cardiomyopathy is far more likely.[2,7,8,21]

Most often seen in postmenopausal women, the clinical presentation of stress-induced cardiomyopathyis is mimicks an acute coronary syndrome with chest pain and EKG abnormality. It is associated with extreme emotional stress such as traffic road accident, financial loss, and other disasters. This myocardial injury has been considered a consequence of intramyocardial calcium overload or ischemic reperfusion phenomenon. Coronary angiogram has revealed the absence of any obstructive coronary artery disease and when performed, cardiac positron emission tomography suggested a metabolic stunned myocardium. Such cardiopulmonary dysfunction is known in many acute neurologic conditions, most commonly described in aneurysmal subarachnoid hemorrhage and intracranial hemorrhage.[11,21]

Neuromuscular causes of cardiac dysfunction have been well recognized. Peripheral nervous disease may be part of a systemic disorder, and that would simultaneously affect the heart. Most striking are the muscle dystrophies, and cardiac involvement may be disproportionately severe. Most are genetic disorders such as Duchenne, Becker's, or Emery-Dreifuss. Myotonic dystrophy may lead to conduction defects and tachyarrhythmias, but seldom to cardiac failure. Anesthetic drugs in these patients may increase the risk of AV blockade. Both facioscapulohumeral and limb-girdle muscular dystrophy have the potential for conduction block abnormalities, but congestive heart failure is less common. Myasthenia gravis is often associated with hyperplasia or tumor (benign or malignant) of the thymus gland. In these patients, the probability of an associated myocarditis is high if cardiac manifestations occur.[16] Myocarditis may present with new arrhythmias such as atrial fibrillation, atrioventricular block, or progressive cardiac failure and ventricular tachycardia.

NEUROGENIC EKG ABNORMALITIES

EKG abnormalities after acute brain injury are nonspecific. The clinical experience is that most of the EKG abnormalities are seen after massive cerebral hemorrhage, aneurysmal subarachnoid hemorrhage, and acute subdural hematoma. These EKG abnormalities include QT prolongation, ST segment changes, and either large, flattened, or inverted T waves.[12,34] Some of these abnormalities predict stress cardiomyopathy. Regional wall motion abnormalities are more common in patients with transient ST segment elevation. Inverted T waves and QT-segment prolongation are more common with left ventricular dysfunction. Prolonged QT interval has been noted after ischemic stroke, and some have suggested it may predict outcome. (The QT interval varies with the heart rate, and a corrected QT [QT_c] is calculated by dividing the QT interval by the square root of the interval between two R waves; normal QT_c is 0.41 seconds in women and 0.39 seconds in men.) QT prolongation is also common in seizures and may be an indirect effect of sympathetic outpouring during seizures.[23] It is known that up to one-third of patients with subarachnoid hemorrhage have prolonged QT time syndrome that may increase the risk of torsades de pointes or ventricular tachycardia.[13,18,33]

ST- and T-wave abnormalities (most commonly T-wave inversions) are most recognizable, but none of these abnormalities predict fatal arrhythmias. Echocardiographic studies have repeatedly shown ventricular dysfunction in these patients.

EKG changes in the early stage of any acute brain injury may also be a predictor of outcome. In subarachnoid hemorrhage (SAH) the combination of tachycardia and prolonged QT interval predicted angiographic vasospasm, but tachycardia and ST segment changes predicted outcome. These associations, albeit interesting, do not satisfactorily explain how these abnormalities connect, and it has been speculated that the link is through a poor cardiac output.[15]

NEUROGENIC CARDIAC ARRHYTHMIAS

There are several factors that can increase the risk of ventricular arrhythmias. The use of vasopressors such as epinephrine and norepinephrine increases the chance for tachyarrhythmias. Atrial fibrillation may be associated with rapid ventricular response. In patients with atrial fibrillation treated with β-blockade, brief discontinuation of β-blockade can cause atrial fibrillation with rapid ventricular response. In some of these patients, this has been prompted by a need to provide permissive hypertension; but this could be at the expense of a sudden increase in ventricular rate with demand ischemia and increasing serum troponins.[17,19,20]

Most dramatic is the propofol infusion syndrome, in which patient's treatment with propofol (mostly for sedation) results in cardiac collapse. Infusions of more than 5 g/kg/h for longer than 48 h increase the risk for the propofol infusion syndrome.[1,28,36] Propofol can cause bradycardia and can decrease myocardial contractility by antagonism of β receptors in calcium channels. Propofol also is associated with excess serum fatty acids that are arrhythmogenic.

In a recent stroke study, coronary artery disease, valvular disease, or hypertensive cardiomyopathy significantly increased the odds of cardiac arrhythmias. The most important ones are hypochloremia and hypomagnesemia, which can lead to QTc interval prolongation.[31] One explanation might be that adrenergic receptors in the heart, when stimulated, can promote repolarization, prolonged QTc, and ventricular arrest. A possible reason for ventricular tachycardia is a peripherally inserted central catheter (PICC). A PICC line is usually inserted in the distal superior vena cava, but improper position into the right ventricle may cause arrhythmias with these central venous catheters.[4]

ANTIARRHYTHMIC DRUGS

For many years, Vaughan Williams/Harrison classification explained action and type (channel or receptor blockade) and varied from class I to class IV

Table 7.1 **Vaughan-Williams Classification of Antiarrhythmic Drugs**

Class	Basic Mechanism	Specifics
I	Sodium-channel blockade	Reduce phase 0 slope and peak of action potential.
II	β-blockade	Block sympathetic activity; reduce rate and conduction.
III	Potassium-channel blockade	Delay repolarization (phase 3) and thereby increase action potential duration and effective refractory period.
IV	Calcium-channel blockade	Block L-type calcium-channels; most effective at SA and AV nodes; reduce rate and conduction.

Abbreviations: APD, action potential duration; ERP, effective refractory period; SA, sinoatrial node; AV, atrioventricular node.

antiarrhythmic drugs (Table 7.1). Class I drugs (lidocaine and mexiletine) are seldom used and have been largely replaced by amiodarone.

Class II drugs are β-blockers and are commonly used on patients who are admitted with prior use of β-blockers. Sudden withdrawal of β-blockers in patients with coronary disease may lead to reflex tachycardia or hypertension. β-blockers may cause insomnia and hallucinations in susceptible neurologic patients. They remain the most important drugs to mute the cardiac arrhythmias associated with catecholamine surge. β-blockers slow AV nodal conduction and slow ventricular response to atrial fibrillation and may reduce demand ischemia due to tachycardia. Labetalol, metoprolol, and esmolol are most commonly used. The half-life of esmolol is minutes, and for most others is 4–5 hours.

The most-used class III drug is amiodarone. It has an antiadrenergic effect and blocks potassium channels. It is now the first drug of choice in patients with ventricular tachycardia and ventricular fibrillation but also slows the ventricular response to atrial fibrillation. The drug has concerning long-term effects (thyroid dysfunction, optic neuritis, peripheral neuropathy, and skin abnormalities) of no concern in acutely ill neurologic patients. Class IV drugs are calcium channel blockers, and of these verapamil or diltiazem are most often used. There is a risk of hypotension due to a potent peripheral vasodilatation when used for control of rapid ventricular response to atrial fibrillation.[19]

Putting It All Together

- The cardiac ventricles have a mostly sympathetic input
- Cardiac arrhythmias are more common in right-sided insula or anterior cingulate lesions

> **BY THE WAY**
> - Atrial fibrillation with new rapid ventricular response is most common
> - Apical ballooning syndrome/stress-induced cardiomyopathy can be a cause of hypotension in any major brain injury
> - Some patients with EKG changes after acute brain injury may have severe coronary artery disease; many do not
> - Echocardiogram in stress cardiomyopathy usually shows regional wall motion abnormalities beyond a single vascular territory

> **NEUROLOGY OF CARDIAC FUNCTION BY THE NUMBERS**
> - ~ 90% of patients with poor-grade SAH have EKG changes
> - ~ 75% of patients with status epilepticus have some cardiac injury
> - ~ 30% of patients with stroke have prolonged QT interval on presentation
> - ~ 25% of patients with acute stroke have cardiac arrhythmias
> - ~ 25% of patients with severe TBI have ventricular arrhythmias
> - ~ 10% of patients with poor-grade SAH have tako-tsubo cardiomyopathy

- Cardiac arrhythmias may be iatrogenic
- Seizures may cause severe bradycardia and arrest
- β-blockade in acute tachyarrhythmias may be needed to protect the heart

References

1. Ahlen K, Buckley CJ, Goodale DB, Pulsford AH. The 'propofol infusion syndrome': the facts, their interpretation and implications for patient care. *Eur J Anaesthesiol* 2006;23:990–998.
2. Akashi YJ, Goldstein DS, Barbaro G, Ueyama T. Takotsubo cardiomyopathy: a new form of acute, reversible heart failure. *Circulation* 2008;118:2754–2762.
3. Armour JA, Ardell JL. *Basic and Clinical Neurocardiology.* Oxford University Press, 2004.
4. Bivins MH, Callahan MJ. Position-dependent ventricular tachycardia related to a peripherally inserted central catheter. *Mayo Clin Proc* 2000;75:414–416.
5. Bolli R, Marbán E. Molecular and cellular mechanisms of myocardial stunning. *Physiol Rev* 1999;79:609–634.
6. Busl KM, Raju M, Ouyang B, Garg RK, Temes RE. Cardiac Abnormalities in Patients with Acute Subdural Hemorrhage. *Neurocrit Care.* 2013;9:79–182.
7. Bybee KA, Prasad A, Barsness GW, et al. Clinical characteristics and thrombolysis in myocardial infarction frame counts in women with transient left ventricular apical ballooning syndrome. *Am J Cardiol* 2004;94:343–346.

8. Bybee KA, Prasad A. Stress-related cardiomyopathy syndromes. *Circulation* 2008;118: 397–409.
9. Caplan LR, Hurst JW. Chimovitz. *Clinical Neurocardiology. Fundamentals and Clinical Cardiology.* New York: CRC Press, 1999.
10. Cheshire WP Jr, Saper CB. The insular cortex and cardiac response to stroke. *Neurology* 2006;66:1296–1297.
11. De Chazal I, Parham WM, Liopyris P, Wijdicks E. Delayed cardiogenic shock and acute lung injury after aneurysmal subarachnoid hemorrhage. *Anesth Analg* 2005; 100:1147–1149.
12. Elrifai AM, Bailes JE, Shih SR, Dianzumba S, Brillman J. Characterization of the cardiac effects of acute subarachnoid hemorrhage in dogs. *Stroke* 1996;27:737–741.
13. Frangiskakis JM, Hravnak M, Crago EA, Tanabe M, Kip KE, Gorcsan J 3rd, et al. Ventricular arrhythmia risk after subarachnoid hemorrhage. *Neurocrit Care* 2009;10:287–294.
14. Fugate JE, Wijdicks EFM, Kumar G, Rabinstein AA. One thing leads to another: GBS complicated by PRES and Takotsubo cardiomyopathy. *Neurocrit Care* 2009;11:395–397.
15. Ibrahim GM, Macdonald RL. Electrographic changes predict angiographic vasospasm after aneurysmal subarachnoid hemorrhage. *Stroke* 2012;43:2102–2107.
16. Joudinaud TM, Fadel E, Thomas-de-Montpreville V, et al. Fatal giant cell myocarditis after thymoma resection in myasthenia gravis. *J Thorac Cardiovasc Surg* 2006;131:494–495.
17. Garg A, Akoum N. Atrial fibrillation and heart failure: beyond the heart rate. *Curr Opin Cardiol* 2013;28:332–336.
18. Khan IA. Long QT syndrome: diagnosis and management. *Am Heart J* 2002;143:7–14.
19. Khoo CW, Lip GY. Acute management of atrial fibrillation. *Chest* 2009;135:849–859.
20. Lee J, Kim K, Lee CC, et al. Low-dose diltiazem in atrial fibrillation with rapid ventricular response. *Am J Emerg Med* 2011;29:849–854.
21. Lee VH, Oh JK, Mulvagh SL, Wijdicks EF. Mechanisms in neurogenic stress cardiomyopathy after aneurysmal subarachnoid hemorrhage. *Neurocrit Care* 2006;5:243–249.
22. Masuda T, Sato K, Yamamoto S, et al. Sympathetic nervous activity and myocardial damage immediately after subarachnoid hemorrhage in a unique animal model. *Stroke* 2002;33:1671–1676.
23. Moseley BD, Wirrell EC, Nickels K, et al. Electrocardiographic and oximetric changes during complex and generalized seizures. *Epilepsy Research* 2011;95: 237–245.
24. Naredi S, Lambert G, Eden E, et al. Increased sympathetic nervous activity in patients with nontraumatic subarachnoid hemorrhage. *Stroke* 2000;31:901–906.
25. Nayate A, Moore SA, Weiss R, et al. Cardiac damage after lesions of the nucleus tractus solitarii. *Am J Physiol Regul Integr Comp Physiol* 2009;296:R272–R279.
26. Novitzky D, Wicomb WN, Cooper KC, Rose AG, Reichart B. Prevention of myocardial injury during brain death by total cardiac sympathectomy in the chacma baboon. *Ann Thorac Surg* 1986;41:520–524.
27. Richard C. Stress-related cardiomyopathies. *Ann Intensive Care* 2011;1:39.
28. Roberts RJ, Barletta JF, Fong JJ, et al. Incidence of propofol-related infusion syndrome in critically ill adults: a prospective, multicenter study. *Crit Care* 2009;13:R169.
29. Ryvlin P, Nashef L, Tomson T. Prevention of sudden unexpected death in epilepsy: a realistic goal? *Epilepsia* 2013;54 Suppl 2:23–28.
30. Samuels MA. The brain-heart connection. *Circulation* 2007;116:77–84.
31. Seet RC, Zhang Y, Rabinstein AA, Wijdicks EFM. Risk factors and consequences of atrial fibrillation with rapid ventricular response in patients with ischemic stroke treated with intravenous thrombolysis. *J Stroke Cerebrovasc Dis* 2013;22: 161–165.
32. Shivalkar B, Van Loon J, Wieland W, et al. Increased intracranial pressure on myocardial structure and function. *Circulation* 1993;87:230–239.
33. Steadt LG, Gilmore RM, Bellolio MF, et al. Prolonged QTc as a predictor of mortality in acute ischemic stroke. *J Stroke Cerebrovascular Dis* 2009:18:308–317.
34. van den Bergh WM, Algra A, Rinkel GJ. Electrocardiographic abnormalities and serum magnesium in patients with subarachnoid hemorrhage. *Stroke* 2004;35:644–648.

35. Wittstein IS, Thierman DR, Lima JA, et al. Neurohumoral features of myocardial stunning due to sudden emotional stress. *N Engl J Med* 2005;352:539–548.
36. Wong JM. Propofol infusion syndrome. *Am J Ther* 2010;17:487–491.
37. Yuki K, Kodama Y, Onda J, Emoto K, Morimoto T, Uozumi T. Coronary vasospasm following subarachnoid hemorrhage as a cause of stunned myocardium. *J Neurosurg* 1991;75:308–311.
39. Zaroff JG, Rordorf GA, Titus JS, et al. Regional myocardial perfusion after experimental subarachnoid hemorrhage. *Stroke* 2000;31:1136–1143.

8

Neurology of Gastroenterology

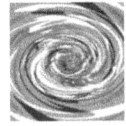

The stomach and gut react to acute brain injury in a predictable way. In the acute phase of brain injury, and in particular when associated with an expanding mass, patients become nauseated and vomit. Acute neurologic signs followed by vomiting in fact are always suggestive of a serious new brain lesion. The sense of hunger disappears in most acutely ill neurologic patients and often when there is a decline of consciousness.

The gut-brain connection has been incompletely understood, but permutations occur simply with the stress of acute brain injury.[13,26] What has been known for decades is that vagal hyperactivity may increase acid production and cause erosions in the fundus and throughout the stomach.[37] Currently, most of the gastric injury can be explained not only by acid but also by local ischemia. There is a sympathoadrenal response releasing angiotensin, constricting the gastric vasculature.[32]

Gastrointestinal mobility is also moderated by neuronal control. Vagal activity increases gastric emptying, and sympathetic activity inhibits mobility. Enteral nutrition is poorly tolerated in severely brain injured patients with very high returns in the acute phase. The colonic loops may also become adynamic (pseudo obstructed) and expand from accumulating gas, which may reach a pressure that can lead to perforation.[14]

One should assume that care requires more than the simple act of inserting a nasogastric tube, placing a feeding order, initiating stress ulcer prophylaxis as part of management of patients on the mechanical ventilator, and providing a bowel regimen. The changed resorption, the changed metabolism, the changed motility, but also the vagally induced injury as a result of suddenly increased intracranial pressure are all issues to be dealt with.

What are the basic recommendations for feeding of the neurologically ill patient? What are the major complications to watch out for? How are motility disturbances treated? How do promotility agents act on the gut? This chapter explains the workings of the gastrointestinal system so that these derangements can be understood.

Principles

Here we will discuss current understanding of brain-gut connection, the possible abnormalities from acute brain injury, and how illness affects nutrition.

THE ANATOMY OF THE GASTROINTESTINAL AUTONOMIC NERVOUS SYSTEM

Both efferent and afferent neurons are distributed throughout the gastrointestinal tract. The gut motility is determined by the vagus nerve, thoracosympathetic nerves, and the S2-S4 nerves.

Although the entire gastrointestinal tract has both extensive sympathetic and parasympathetic innervation, most upper gastrointestinal motility is controlled by the parasympathetic vagus nerve.[18,33] The vagus nerve increases mobility and gastric acid production. The multiple vagus nerve fibers originating from the nucleus ambiguus target the larynx and esophagus, and the dorsal motor nucleus of the vagus targets the stomach until the descending colon. The distal colon and rectum receive input from the sacral spinal cord. (Figure 8.1).[18,33] Vagal and sacral nerves carry parasympathetic fibers responsible for basic function (excitatory), but the splanchnic nerves carry inhibitory sympathetic fibers. The neurotransmitter within the sympathetic system is norepinephrine, which inhibits acetylcholine release, blocking excitatory pathways. The sympathetic input—branched off the prevertebral sympathetic ganglia—is thus inhibitory in the gut and excitatory in the sphincter.[15,16]

There are many automated responses such as the peristaltic reflex, and many intrinsic pacemakers in the gastric greater curvature and in the duodenal bulb. These intrinsic primary afferent neurons form a submucosal and myenteric plexus.[15,16] The pacemakers are part of an "electric mesh" of neurons, and the vagus nerve synapses with these hardwired circuits, but peristalsis is possible after denervation. The neurotransmitters associated with these synaptic circuits are most commonly acetylcholine, but there are many more. Several others have been identified and also include a vasoactive interstitial polypeptide that causes vasodilatation and glandular secretion. It has also been discovered that the gut is an endocrine organ. Cholecystokinin (CCK) acts on the vagus nerve, resulting in a relaxing response reducing gastric emptying. The "endocrine failure" in critical illness and delayed gastric emptying is explained by the suppression of some of these hormones.

Continence is maintained due to parasympathetic sacral input leading to contraction of the puborectalis. One important reflex mechanism is the vagovagal reflex. A vagal excitatory (muscarinic) pathway maintains gastric tone, and a vagal inhibitory pathway relaxes the stomach. The information from mechanical deformation or from humeral factors or other chemicals is relayed to the brainstem and spinal cord through vagal and spinal afferents.

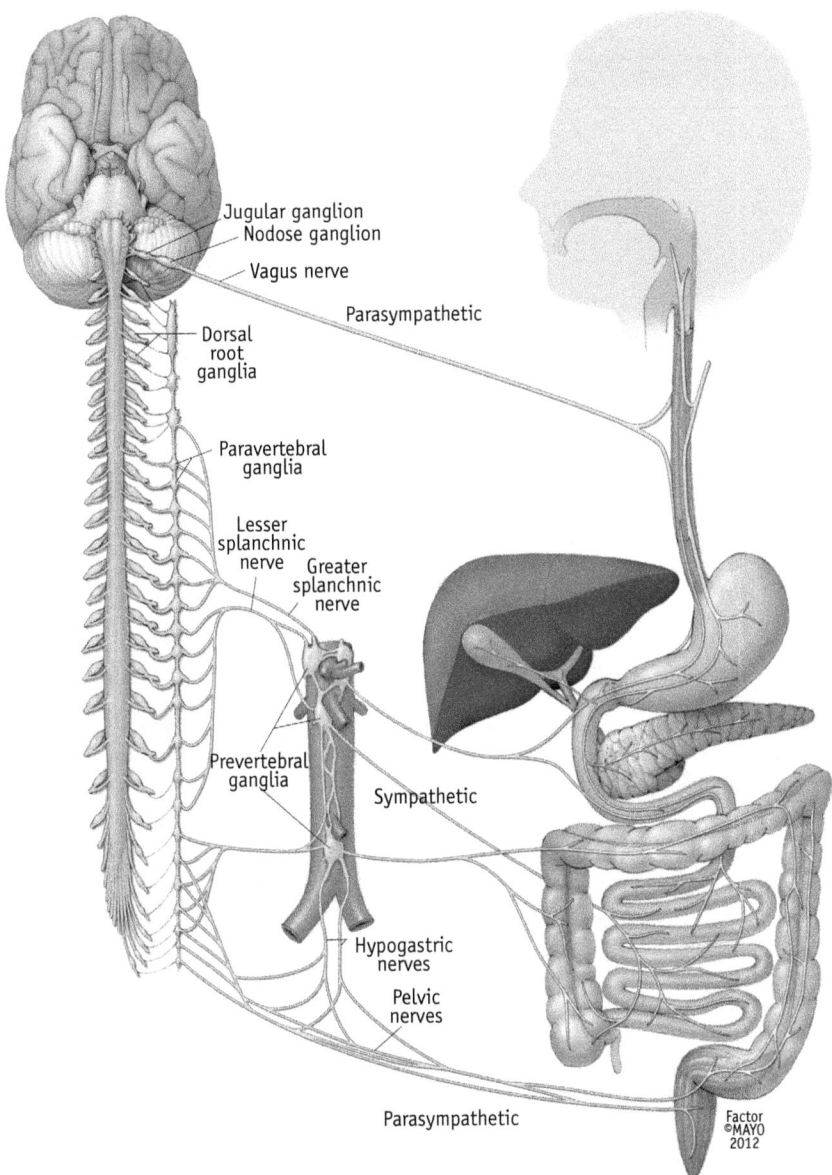

Figure 8.1 Sympathetic and parasympathetic input and gut-to-brain connection.

The functions of the gastrointestinal system that may become impaired are mainly secretion and motility and are all directly under control of the autonomic nervous system. Secretion in the gastrointestinal tract is needed for digestion, and motility is needed for transport and absorption of nutrients. Neuroendocrine signals may result in hunger (ghrelin), nausea (5-HT), or satiety (glucagon-like peptide, peptide YY).[2,4,10,29,36,42] Gut sensations are a result of the activation of the

Table 8.1 **Gastrointestinal Hormones**

Substance	Function	In illness
Ghrelin[4,35,39]	• Appetite stimulant • Gastric emptying	Decreased critical illness
Motilin[37]	• Gastric emptying • Increases stomach contractions	Erythromycin increases motilin Hyperglycemia decreases motilin
Cholecystokinin[16,28]	• Contraction gallbladder • Appetite decrease	Early enteral nutrition blunts secretion
Peptide YY[16]	• Reduces gastric emptying • Inhibits appetite	Increased in critical illness
Glucagon-like peptide (GLP-1)[5,7]	• Reduces hyperglycemia • Reduces gastric emptying	Improves stress-induced hyperglycemia

insula and orbitofrontal cortex connecting and signaling the anterior cingulate cortex (Table 8.1).[26]

NEUROGASTROENTEROLOGY

Gastric injury is due to the effects of acid. The vulnerability of the mucosa may be increased by substances such as acetylcholine, histamine, and endogenous thyrotropin-releasing hormone.[12] Disruption of the mucus gel overlying the gastric epithelium may also be a consequence of previous bile reflux, uremia, alcohol, aspirin, and nonsteroidal anti-inflammatory drugs. Another major effect is hypoperfusion resulting in diminished mucus production and compromise of the mucus barrier, exposing the epithelial layer to acidic material. Intestinal motility is impaired in any patient with bed rest and exacerbated by any type of stress, thus, patients rapidly become constipated.

Gastrointestinal motility is a major defense mechanism against infection of the gut and needs to be maintained.[9] Outcome studies in patients with severe strokes and head injury suggest that early nutritional support reduced mortality and incidence of nosocomial infections.[43] Enterally fed patients have better immune function, fewer infectious complications, and less sepsis. How the gut becomes immobile in some patients is explained by sympathetic effects (inhibition and no contraction) and parasympathetic effects (excitation and no relaxation). When the splanchnic efferents are stimulated, the tone and intestinal movements decline (splanchnicectomy prevents ileus). Support for a sympathetic overdrive comes from clinical improvement using adrenergic blockers and the acetylcholinesterase inhibitor neostigmine. Peripheral opioid receptors may also pick up endogenous opioids or administered opioids and immobilize the colon. Gastroparesis may also result from severe hypokalemia, hypoadrenocorticism, diabetes mellitus, uremia, drugs (anticholinergics, β-adrenergic agonists, opiates), and acute abdominal inflammation.[8,11]

Knowing the anatomy, it is now possible to understand the working action of certain drugs that improve motility. For example, in addition to its dopaminergic properties, metoclopramide also possesses $5HT_4$ receptor and $5HT_3$ receptor antagonism. Opioid receptors—μ-receptor subtype—are widespread throughout the enteric nervous system; activation delays gastric emptying, increases segmental contractions, and reduces propulsive contractions.[17,18,19,20]

Impaired gastrointestinal motility has been demonstrated in critically ill patients receiving opioids and may play a large role in the morbidity associated with gastroparesis. Intravenous naloxone administration has been associated with increased gastric emptying. Enteral naloxone blocks intestinal opioid receptors in the gut, but it is poorly absorbed systemically because of its first-pass hepatic metabolism. This should still allow oral administration of naloxone or other opioid antagonists to selectively block gastrointestinal receptors while leaving systemic effects intact. Improved motility has indeed been observed in patients receiving opioids treated with oral naloxone.

Erythromycin is a macrolide antibiotic that increases gastrointestinal motility by acting on motilin receptors in smooth-muscle cells of the stomach (motilin receptors are located on cholinergic nerves).[21,22,25] The prokinetic dose of erythromycin is much lower than the antimicrobial dose. Ranitidine and nizatidine are known histaminergic H-2 receptor antagonists for regulation of gastric acid secretion, but they also inhibit acetylcholinesterase within the enteric nervous system.[42] Decreased acetylcholinesterase at the neuromuscular junction enhances the effects of acetylcholine on muscarinic cholinergic smooth-muscle receptors and smooth-muscle contraction.

EFFECTS OF ILLNESS ON NUTRITION

Integrity of the gastrointestinal tract is largely dependent on enteral feeding. Enteral feeding not only stimulates cellular proliferation but also maintains enzyme function and normal villus height. There are several endogenous agents that have a major trophic effect on the epithelium.

The gut flora, with over 500 aerobic and anaerobic species, prevent pathogenic microorganisms from entry; however, stress, illness, immunosuppression, and, most importantly, antibiotic regimens change the equation. Changes may also increase expression of so-called virulence genes in bacteria. The mucosae immune system, located in the gut lymphoid follicles, is another line of defense. Sepsis may destroy the mucosal immune system.

If the gut is not fed, bacterial overgrowth may occur and may challenge the mucosal defenses. There is rapidly decreasing mucosal mass, loss of villus height, and eventually villus atrophy in patients who have been treated with parenteral nutrition for a prolonged period of time. This will all lead to increased permeability and eventually systemic endotoxemia. Continuous enteral feeding will not only maintain the microbial flora in the gastrointestinal tract but also will have a significant impact on immunological response associated with infections.[35,37]

There is reason to believe that immune suppression may play a role in microbial overgrowth. There is significant interest in immunonutrition and using immune-enhancing diets. This includes the use of L-arginine, which may stimulate wound healing; omega-3 fatty acids, which could reduce platelet aggregation, reduce blood clotting, and also would reduce the appearance of proinflammatory cytokines; and L-glutamine, which is used by epithelial cells; but none of these supplements have improved outcome. Similar data have shown that antioxidants, vitamins, and trace minerals have not proven to be beneficial in critically ill patients.

In Practice

Early feeding of the gut to guarantee adequate nutrition is part of daily care.[3] The main goal of nutrition should be to preserve muscle mass, and to provide adequate fluids, minerals, and fats.

BASICS OF NUTRITION

There is a fundamental difference between starvation and the much more common hypermetabolic state. In starvation, the major physiologic changes are characterized by decreased energy expenditure and utilization of alternative fuel sources. Patients can tolerate extended periods of semistarvation because the body responds to decreased energy intake by reduction of the basal metabolic rate and favors a state in which the fat supplies are used as primary fuel.

Patients with a neurologic catastrophe respond differently.[6,23,43] The metabolic rate is dramatically increased (hypermetabolism); and rather than depletion of fat, protein stores from lean body mass–muscle mostly–are rapidly mobilized. The major physiologic changes that are characterized by increased metabolic rate are, leukocytosis, hyperglycemia, hypoalbuminemia, and increased blood urea nitrogen.

Caloric needs can be estimated by weight and approximate 25 to 30 kcal/kg per day. The Harris-Benedict formulas, however, are more accurate in determining caloric needs. Nutritional needs in patients with neurologic critical illness should be calculated with the Harris-Benedict equation to obtain the basal energy expenditure (BEE) in calories. The Harris-Benedict formulas are based on kilograms of weight (W), centimeters of height (H), and years of age (A). For men, the formula is BEE = $66.5 + 13.8W + 5H - 6.8A$, and for women,

BEE = 655 + 9.6W + 1.8H − 4.7A. This method, although introduced in healthy persons, remains the most practical means of obtaining daily caloric needs. Correcting factors for specific critical disease states, which primarily add a certain percentage to the calculated value, have been proposed, but they increase the inaccuracy of an estimate. More specifically, no correcting factors are known in acute brain injury. It is, however, common practice to add a "stress factor" in patients with an acute central nervous system catastrophic event and marked sympathetic manifestations, such as profuse sweating, hyperthermia, hypertension, and tachycardia. (Total calories are then calculated as BEE plus 20%.) In obese patients, 75% of the basal Harris-Benedict calculation based on obese weight seems reasonable. The estimated energy expenditure subsequently is divided into proteins of 1.5 g/kg per day, and the remaining calories are evenly divided between carbohydrates and lipids. Enteral products in the formulary usually contain 1 kcal/1 mL. In obese patients, nutritional requirements mostly involve hypocaloric high protein nutrition in patients with a BMI over 27. The simplest way to monitor nutritional support, however, is to weigh patients regularly.

Malnutrition should be recognized in emergency admission of patients with severe traumatic brain injury or fulminant meningitis, conditions that are more prevalent in alcoholics and patients with illegal drug use. Malnutrition may impair respiratory muscles, decrease respiratory drive, and diminish the lung defense mechanism. Vitamin B_1 (thiamine) deficiency might lead to development of Wernicke-Korsakoff syndrome (confusional state, horizontal and vertical nystagmus, gaze palsy, and ataxia of gait). Intravenous administration of thiamine (50 mg IV initially and then 50–100 mg daily for 5 to 7 days) prevents development of Wernicke-Korsakoff syndrome after carboxyhydrate loads.

The integrity of the gut is maintained by enteral feeding and greatly challenged by parenteral nutrition. It is prudent to consider postpyloric feeding in patients with neurological catastrophes, because gastric atony increases the risk of aspiration. However, drug absorption in the jejunum may be unreliable. Enteral feeding should preferably be done by continuous infusion with a volumetric pump. Current protocols recommend starting feeding at 25 mL/h and increasing the volume by 25 mL/h every 4 hours until the goal of nutrition is achieved. When a gastric residual volume is more than 250 mL, feeding should be held for 4 hours and then restarted at the same rate but with more gradual increase. Problems with enteral feedings are frequent, and include diarrhea, nausea, and abdominal distension.

Gastrostomy placement should be considered in patients with prolonged needs for enteral nutrition due to impairment in swallowing mechanisms. This placement should be considered if recovery of dysphagia is not anticipated for 2–3 weeks (more details on nutrition are found in the volume *Providing Acute Care*).

GASTROINTESTINAL COMPLICATIONS AFTER BRAIN INJURY

Clinically, physicians taking care of acute neurologic disease are confronted with either gastrointestinal bleeding or serious motility problems—some that are iatrogenic in nature. Two conditions are discussed in more detail.

Gastrointestinal Hemorrhage

Most of the injury can be explained by a combination of local ischemia and acid. Blood flow may be compromised by marked episodes of hypotension—for example, in patients with polytrauma—and increased parasympathetic nervous system activation through the vagus nerve plays a crucial role.

The currently accepted mechanism is that the sympathetic nervous system stimulates, with the adrenal gland prompting release of angiotensin constricting the gastric vasculature. Therefore, hypoperfusion and diminished mucous production and compromise of the mucous barrier expose the gastric lining to acidic material. Patients with severe traumatic brain injury or spinal cord injury—and any postoperative patient—are at risk. The use of high doses of corticosteroids may be a factor.

Gastrointestinal hemorrhage from "stress erosions" are much less common. Cushing was one of the first clinicians who described an ulcer (and perforation) in the stomach as a result of an acute brain injury (in his case, posterior fossa tumor surgery was the most common cause). These ulcers are due to a different pathophysiology but associated with major physical and thermal trauma, shock or sepsis, and even mechanical ventilation alone as stressors.

Prophylactic acid suppression is commonly instituted and after an era of histamine-2 receptor antagonists, proton pump inhibitors became a preferred treatment to protect patients at higher risk for acute brain injury–induced gastric ulcers and gastric hemorrhage.[1,24]

Drugs are commonly used to reduce gastric acid secretion, but the incidence of bleeding is so low that it does not warrant indiscriminate use of prophylaxis in general ward patients. It is clear that over one hundred patients will have to be treated to prevent one transfusion-required gastric hemorrhage. Many physicians agree that early enteral feeding is the best protection against stress ulcer syndrome. Major risk factors for critically ill patients include mechanical ventilation of more than 2 days, coagulopathy, shock, sepsis, severe burns defined as more than 30% of body surface, and multiorgan failure. Tailoring stress prophylaxis to these high-risk patients makes perfect sense. Histamine-2 receptor antagonists are usually initiated as part of the ventilator bundle because they effectively reduce stress-related bleeding and do not increase nosocomial pneumonia. However, histamine-2 receptor antagonists in susceptible patients (elderly, prior dementia, prior renal and liver disease) may cause acute agitation and hallucinations. It may also cause gradual (but not severe) thrombocytopenia.

Proton pump inhibitors (PPIs; omeprazole, lansoprazole) bind to the hydrogren potassium ATPase, and this stops secreting acid into the stomach. The problems with PPIs have been well recognized and include administration (time-consuming preparation dissolving the drug in sodium bicarbonate; clogging feeding tubes), costs (higher than other prophylactic drugs), and higher risk of *Clostridium difficile* infection. Another commonly identified problem is that many patients stay on prophylaxis long after acute illness has passed.[28]

The evaluation of stress-related mucosal bleeding is first to determine source of bleeding. It may be difficult to be certain, and bleeding may come from oral site or tracheostomy. This may require urgent endoscopy if the patient continues to hemorrhage despite blood transfusion and adequate volume resuscitation.

Endoscopic findings are useful and may predict bleeding risk. The Forrest grade is typically used: Forrest grade IA = arterial bleeding; Forrest grade Forrest IB = oozing; Forrest grade IIA = nonbleeding vessel visible; IIB = adherent clot; Forrest grade IIC = flat-pigmented clot; Forrest grade III = clean ulcer base. The Forrest grade predicts the chance of rebleeding, which is 90% with showing active arterial bleeding which decreases to 50% if there is a nonbleeding vessel visible and is 5% at grade III. Endoscopic treatment is warranted with Forrest I and IIa ulcers.[24]

Repeat endoscopic procedure is not useful after the patient has been adequately treated.[24] Intravenous PPIs are initiated after a bolus injection. Angiography with the opportunity to proceed to intra-arterial embolization is rarely needed, but very effective. A transfusion requirement of more than 8 units in 24 hours is one frequently used criterion, but this depends on what hemoglobin level triggers a transfusion.[24] Recent evidence in a general critically ill population argues for moderation and transfusing at 7 g/dL, but this level may be too low in critically ill neurologic patients.[39]

Gastric Immobility

Gastric immobility is linked to mechanical ventilation, and the frequency may increase in patients with increased intracranial pressure or spinal cord injury.[30] Gastric motility disorders may be specifically due to esophageal malfunction and premorbid conditions such as diabetes, alcoholism, or systemic illness, but benzodiazepines and opioids also contribute greatly.[8,27] Gastric emptying may be reduced from hyperglycemia that reduces vagal efferent activity.

The major motility syndrome is adynamic ileus of the colon (Ogilvie syndrome) presenting as abdominal distension or abdominal pain, and may result in either no stool or diarrhea. Duration of distension and cecal diameter (more than 9 cm) is associated with a higher risk of cecal perforation. Clinicians should very much be aware that many drugs in the ICU cause motility disturbances. Opioids do cause constipation and inhibit gastrointestinal transmission even in small doses. Other drugs that do the same but are typically not considered are clonidine, dexmedetomidine, dopamine, and paracetamol.

Table 8.2 **Effect of Motility Drugs**

Drug	Stomach	Small Bowel	Colon
Cisapride	+	+	o
Domperidone	+	o	+
Erythromycin	++	+	o
Metoclopramide	+	+	o
Neostigmine	o	o	+

Intestinal motility disorders are best treated with cisapride, metoclopramide, neostigmine, or domperidone. The drugs are shown in Table 8.2, but the degree of improvement may not be throughout the entire gastrointestinal tract. The effect of a single dose of neostigmine can be rapid and dramatic and is preferred. Prior use of opioids may also direct treatment; and thus opioid antagonist methylnaltrexone is often used, because it does not cross the blood-brain barrier and, therefore, does not counter the analgesic effect of opioids.[14]

Putting It All Together

- Vagal function moves the gut; sympathetic input stops the gut
- Motility disorders are common, but are commonly effectively treated with neostigmine
- Early gut feeding reduces bacterial overgrowth
- Many patients are underfed and need 20% additional calories to account for stress
- Gastrointestinal hemorrhage can be prevented by prophylaxis. Blood transfusion after GI bleeding is very uncommon after acute brain injury
- Endoscopy determines risk for rebleeding

BY THE WAY

- Metoclopramide is a serotonergic agonist and D_2-dopaminergic antagonist
- Cisapride is a serotonergic agonist
- Erythromycin is serotonergic agonist and a motilin agonist
- Naloxone blocks intestinal opioid receptors
- Ranitidine is a acetylcholinesterase inhibitor and a muscarinic agonist
- Neostigmine is a cholinergic agonist

GASTROENTEROLOGY BY THE NUMBERS
- ~90% of patients with severe brain injury need a gastrostomy
- ~80% of patients with spinal cord injury develop gut motility disorders
- ~50% of patients with severe brain injury develop gut motility disorders
- ~50% loss of mucosal mass with no feeding
- ~20% of critically ill patients are underfed
- ~20% of patients with severe brain injury may have poor calorie intake
- ~10% of patients with severe brain injury will be malnourished on admission
- ~5% of patients with severe brain injury have a gastric bleeding

References

1. Alhazzani W, Alenezi F, Jaeschke RZ, et al. Proton pump inhibitors versus histamine 2 receptor antagonists for stress prophylaxis in critically ill patients: a systemic review and meta-analysis. *Crit Care Med* 2013;41:1555–1564.
2. Baynes KC, Dhillo WS, Bloom SR. Regulation of food intake by gastrointestinal hormones. *Curr Opin Gastroenterol* 2006;22:626–631.
3. Behara AS, Peterson SJ, Chen Y, Butsch J, Lateef O, Komanduri S. Nutrition support in the critically ill: a physician survey. *J Parenter Enteral Nutr* 32:113–119, 2008.
4. Broglio F, Arvat E, Benso A, et al. Ghrelin, a natural GH secretagogue produced by the stomach, induces hyperglycemia and reduces insulin secretion in humans. *J Clin Endocrinol Metab* 2001;86:5083–5086.
5. Burcelin R. The gut-brain axis: a major glucoregulatory player. *Diabetes Metab* 2010;36:S54–58.
6. Cerra FB, Benitez MR, Blackburn GL, et al. Applied nutrition in ICU patients: a consensus statement of the American College of Chest Physicians. *Chest* 1997;111:769–778.
7. Chapman MJ, Fraser RJ, Matthews G, et al. Glucose absorption and gastric emptying in critical illness. *Crit Care* 2009;13:R140.
8. Chapman MJ, Nguyen NQ, Deane AM. Gastrointestinal dysmotility: clinical consequences and management of the critically ill patient. *Gastroenterol Clin North Am* 2011;40:725–739.
9. Daneman R, Rescigno M. The gut immune barrier and the blood-brain barrier: are they so different? *Immunity* 2009;31:722–735.
10. Deane A, Chapman MJ, Fraser RJ, Horowitz M. Bench-to-bedside review: the gut as an endocrine organ in the critically ill. *Crit Care* 2010;14:228.
11. Dive A, Foret F, Jamart J, Bulpa P, Installé E. Effect of dopamine on gastrointestinal motility during critical illness. *Intensive Care Med* 2000;26:901–907.
12. Duerksen DR. Stress-related mucosal disease in critically ill patients. *Best Pract Res Clin Gastroenterol* 2003;17:327–344.
13. Fetissov SO, Déchelotte P. The new link between gut-brain axis and neuropsychiatric disorders. *Curr Opin Clin Nutr Metab Care* 2011;14:477–482.
14. Fruhwald S, Holzer P, Metzler H. Intestinal motility disturbances in intensive care patients pathogenesis and clinical impact. *Intensive Care Med* 2007;33:36–44.
15. Furness JB. Types of neurons in the enteric nervous system. *J Auton Nerv Syst* 2000:81:87–96.
16. Furness, JB. *The Enteric Nervous System*. Blackwell, Oxford, 2006.
17. Gershon MD. Review article: serotonin receptors and transporters—roles in normal and abnormal gastrointestinal motility. *Aliment Pharmacol Ther* 2004;20:3–14.
18. Goyal RK, Hirano J. The enteric nervous system. *N Engl J Med* 1996;334:1106–1115.

19. Grundy D. Signalling the state of the digestive tract. *Auton Neurosci* 2006;125:76–80.
20. Heyland DK, Tougas G, King D, Cook DJ. Impaired gastric emptying in mechanically ventilated, critically ill patients. *Intensive Care Med* 1996;22:1339–1344.
21. Janssens J, Peeters TL, Vantrappen G, et al. Improvement of gastric emptying in diabetic gastroparesis by erythromycin: preliminary studies. *N Engl J Med* 1990;322:1028–1031.
22. Jones KL, Berry M, Kong MF, et al. Hyperglycemia attenuates the gastrokinetic effect of erythromycin and affects the perception of postprandial hunger in normal subjects. *Diabetes Care* 1999;22:339–344.
23. Kao CH, Ho YJ, Changlai SP, Ding HJ. Gastric emptying in spinal cord injury patients. *Dig Dis Sci* 1999;44:1512–1515.
24. Lau JY, Barkun A, Fan DM, Kuipers EJ, Yang YS, Chan FK. Challenges in the management of acute peptic ulcer bleeding. *Lancet*. 2013;381:2033–2043.
25. MacLaren R, Kiser TH, Fish DN, Wischmeyer PE. Erythromycin vs metoclopramide for facilitating gastric emptying and tolerance to intragastric nutrition in critically ill patients. *JPEN J Parenter Enteral Nutr* 2008;32:412–419.
26. Mayer EA. Gut feelings: the emerging biology of gut-brain communication. *Nat Rev Neurosci* 2011;12:453–466.
27. Meier JJ. Waking up the gut in critically ill patients. *Crit Care* 2010;14:183.
28. Murphy CE, Stevens AM, Ferrentino N, et al. Frequency of inappropriate continuation of acid suppressive therapy after discharge in patients who began therapy in the surgical intensive care unit. *Pharmacotherapy* 2008;28:968–976.
29. Nguyen NQ, Fraser RJ, Bryant LK, et al. The relationship between gastric emptying, plasma cholecystokinin, and peptide YY in critically ill patients. *Crit Care* 2007;11:R132.
30. Nguyen NQ, Ng MP, Chapman M, Fraser RJ, Holloway RH. The impact of admission diagnosis on gastric emptying in critically ill patients. *Crit Care* 2007;11:R16.
31. Pilichiewicz AN, Chaikomin R, Brennan IM, et al. Load-dependent effects of duodenal glucose on glycemia, gastrointestinal hormones, antropyloroduodenal motility, and energy intake in healthy men. *Am J Physiol Endocrinol Metab* 2007;293:E743–E753.
32. Puleo F, Arvanitakis M, Van Gossum A, Preiser JC. Gut failure in the ICU. *Semin Respir Crit Care Med* 2011;32:626–638.
33. Ratcliffe EM, Farrar NR, Fox EA. Development of the vagal innervation of the gut: steering the wandering nerve. *Neurogastroenterol Motil* 2011;23:898–911.
34. Rauch S, Krueger K, Turan A, Roewer N, Sessler DI. Determining small intestinal transit time and pathomorphology in critically ill patients using video capsule technology. *Intensive Care Med* 2009;35:1054–1059.
35. Rhee SH, Pothoulakis C, Mayer EA. Principles and clinical implications of the brain-gut-enteric microbiota axis. *Nat Rev Gastroenterol Hepatol* 2009;6:306–314.
36. Tack J, Depoortere I, Bisschops R, et al. Influence of ghrelin on gastric emptying and meal-related symptoms in idiopathic gastroparesis. *Aliment Pharmacol Ther* 2005;22:847–853.
37. Thompson JS. The intestinal response to critical illness. *Am J Gastroenterol* 1995;90:190–200.
38. Vantrappen G, Janssens J, Peeters TL, et al. Motilin and the interdigestive migrating motor complex in man. *Dig Dis Sci* 1979;24:497–500.
39. Villaneuva C, Colomo A, Bosch A. Transfusion strategies for upper gastrointestinal bleeding. *New Engl J Med* 2013;378:11–21
40. Wren AM, Seal LJ, Cohen MA, et al. Ghrelin enhances appetite and increases food intake in humans. *J Clin Endocrinol Metab* 2001;86:5992.
41. Young B, Ott L, Yingling B, et al: Nutrition and brain injury. *J Neurotrauma* 1992;9 Suppl 1:S375–S383.
42. Zac-Varghese S, Tan T, Bloom SR. Hormonal interactions between gut and brain. *Discov Med* 2010;10:543–552.
43. Zarbock SD, Steinke D, Hatton J, Magnuson B, Smith KM, Cook AM. Successful enteral nutritional support in the neurocritical care unit. *Neurocrit Care* 2008;9:210–216.

9

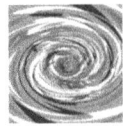

Neurology of the Bladder

Micturition is under the control of the central and peripheral nervous system, and a well-timed mechanism exists. The frontal cortex and pons are involved with voluntary control, and lesions in these locations result in uninhibited bladder contractions. The brain areas that are involved in the regulation of urine storage have been elucidated largely as a result of functional MRI studies, but most neural circuits are unknown and hypothetical.[23] Spinal cord lesions are usually associated with an acute detrusor areflexia. Storage and micturition reflexes may become abnormal, a condition best known as neurogenic bladder.

Voiding difficulties and urinary incontinence after acute central nervous system injury are so common that they may be taken for granted.[33] Most patients will receive an indwelling catheter, and for many of us bladder management may arguably stop there. Even more embarrassing, only one in four physicians in teaching hospitals know whether their patients have an urinary catheter.[45] Furthermore, in the management of bladder dysfunction, it is often not realized that bladder symptoms are treatable—perhaps the most treatable of neurologic deficits—but are also usually ignored in assessment of the patient (e.g., major stroke scales do not measure incontinence).[36,38]

Understanding the basic neurourology of control of the bladder and its pharmacology has been a conundrum for many physicians, but some knowledge is necessary because good treatment options are available.[13,21,23,24]

Urgent questions are: What is a urologic emergency in acutely ill neurologic patients? What voiding disorders need to be recognized? How can we best provide bladder care? How do we maintain continence? This chapter reviews current clinically relevant concepts of micturition and bladder function. Because spinal cord injury and bladder dysfunction are closely linked, this topic is reviewed in more detail.

Principles

There are central nervous system pathways involving micturition as well as specialized areas of the brain, spinal cord, and peripheral ganglia.[7,16,22] Specific neurons for micturition include the neurons of Barrington's nucleus (better known

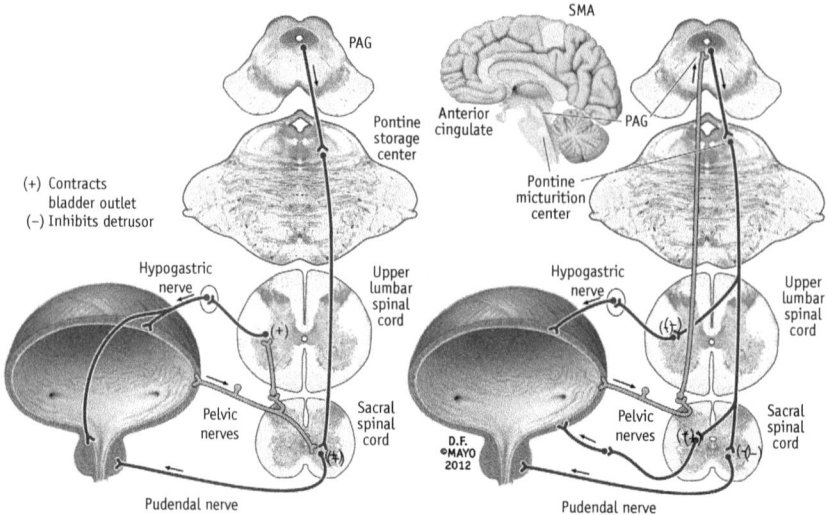

Figure 9.1 Pathways associated with bladder emptying.

as the pontine micturition center), neurons in the periaqueductal gray, neurons in the caudal and preoptic hypothalamus, and neurons in the cerebral cortex, particularly in the medial frontal cortex.[5,23] As expected, owing to its role in executing plans, the anterior cingulate cortex plays an important role.[27,30] It receives signals from the detrusor muscle of the bladder—starting with a bladder volume of approximately 400 mL—and then the anterior cingulate cortex decides whether to void or to contract the urethral sphincter that holds voiding. The prefrontal cortex is also involved in timing of voiding (to go now or later) and has a link with the periaqueductal gray matter and, therefore, could suppress voiding when willfully desired.[6]

The pontine micturition center apparently has a mechanism that can switch between storage and voiding. Storage occurs by inhibition of parasympathetic activity, which relaxes the detrusor muscle of the bladder wall. In addition, tonic constriction of the urethral sphincters, mediated by sympathetic and pudendal nerves, maintains continence.

Bladder voiding could work as follows: activation of the pontine and micturition center results in urethral relaxation, activation of the parasympathetic efferents, contraction of the bladder, increase in intravesical pressure, and urination.[3]

Bladder relaxation is due to activation of the parasympathetic pathway to the urethra. It is still uncertain if voluntary voiding is the result of interruption of the tonic suppression by the prefrontal cortex of the periaqueductal gray input to the pontine micturition center—a truly let-go mechanism (Figure 9.1).

The peripheral innervation of the bladder, urethra, and sphincters consists anatomically of both the sympathetic innervation from thoracolumbar (T-11, L-2) spinal cord and the parasympathetic innervation originating off the lower

9. Neurology of the Bladder   119

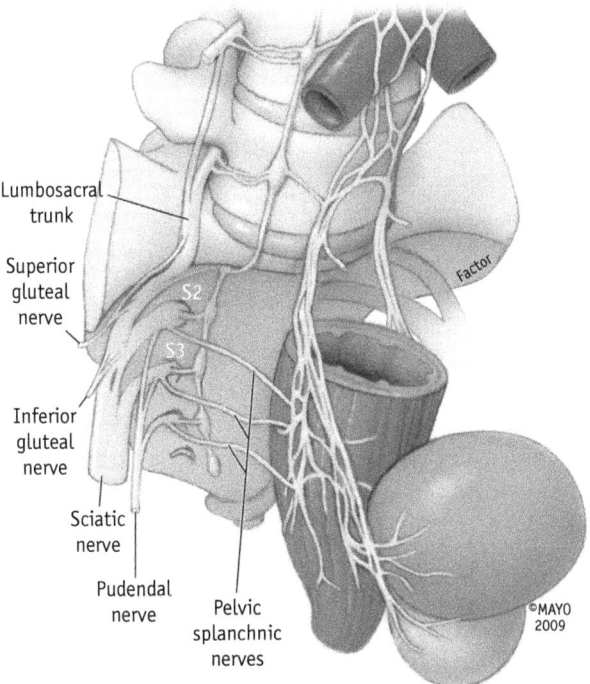

Figure 9.2 Innervation of Bladder.

sacral segments (S3-S4) of the spinal cord (Figure 9.2).[49] These two systems are tightly coordinated. The sympathetic fibers originate in the segments of the spinal cord and then travel through the inferior mesenteric ganglia and the hypogastric nerve, or through the paravertebral chain to enter the pelvic nerves at the base of the bladder and urethra.

The lower urinary tract, with the bladder and urethra, has a major role in storage of urine and voiding. The parasympathetic postganglionic nerve fibers trigger the human bladder, resulting in the detrusor contraction and urinary flow. The parasympathetic nerves of the sacral segment S2—through the pudendal nerve—also provide the fibers for voluntary control of the external sphincters. The parasympathetic nerves also cause erections, and thus in peripheral lesions lack of detrusor contractility is coupled with inability to achieve an erection. Conversely, spontaneous erections (priapism) occur at the moment of acute spinal cord injury. It is seen mostly in complete acute spinal cord lesions and at any level due to the low sacral origin of the parasympathetic fibers. It occurs usually at the time of injury or very soon thereafter as a result of acute severance of the sympathetic input resulting in unopposed parasympathetic input.

To summarize in more detail: a normal micturition trigger involves filling of the bladder, slow rise of pressure, increased urethral resistance, and no cholinergic output. When the micturition threshold is reached, the sympathetic nerves fire and contract the internal sphincter. The external sphincter is also in a contracted state through the pudendal nerve. Voluntary desire to void will release the sympathetic activity and decrease the sphincter resistance, resulting in urinary flow. Thus, voiding is stimulation of parasympathetics, inhibition of the sympathetics, and inhibition of the somatic nerves to the urogenital sphincter. Filling and storage are the opposite. Normally, we start to sense bladder filling at 100 mL and voiding desire around 300–500 mL. At 2 L many of us will become restless or agitated.

How is bladder function abnormal in neurologic disease? Neurologic causes of bladder dysfunction can be categorized as suprapontine, infrapontine, or infrasacral. The distinguishing characteristics are shown in Table 9.1. Impaired detrusor contractions can be due to reduced parasympathetic drive from the bulbospinal pathway, and cauda equina lesions can affect the sacral pathway, resulting in voiding dysfunction, typically because of nonrelaxing sphincters and poorly sustained detrusor contractions.[4]

A general rule of thumb is that suprapontine lesions lead to detrusor hyperreflexia, also known as an overactive bladder, but without detrusor sphincter dyssynergia. With detrusor sphincter dyssynergia, the sphincter tightens during contraction intermittently, and this is therefore very different from the normal relaxation during bladder contraction. The major conditions that cause urinary incontinence are ischemic stroke, acute spinal cord injury, and acute cauda equina syndrome.

In most instances, frontal lobe lesions, typically in the setting of stroke, brain tumor, hydrocephalus, and subdural hematoma, may produce urinary symptoms such as urinary incontinence and urgency. Detrusor hyperreflexia has been seen with acute lesions of the frontal lobe and basal ganglia, but there may also be inhibited sphincter relaxation with these lesions. Patients with ischemic stroke

Table 9.1 **Diagnostic Evaluation of Neurologic Bladder Dysfunction**

	Suprapontine Lesion (e.g., Frontal Lobe)	*Infrapontine Suprasacral Lesion (e.g., Spinal Cord)*	*Infrasacral Lesion (e.g., Conus Medullaris, Cauda Equina)*
Symptoms:	Urgency, increased frequency	Urgency, increased frequency	Hesitancy, retention
Bladder scan	No postvoid residual urine	Postvoid residual urine	Postvoid residual urine
Uroflowmetry	Normal flow	Interrupted flow	Poor/absent flow
Urodynamics	Detrusor overactivity	Detrusor overactivity, detrusor–sphincter dyssynergia	Detrusor underactivity, sphincter insufficiency

Modified from reference 34.

have incontinence when the lesion is located in the anterior medial frontal lobe and putamen.

Many chronic and degenerative neurologic diseases cause urologic dysfunction. Patients may develop acute neurologic complications in the setting of Parkinson's disease, multisystem atrophy or multiple sclerosis.[17] Parkinson's disease is associated with frequent urinary tract symptoms and correlates with the severity of the disease. Patients with Parkinson's disease usually have an overactive bladder and frequent nocturia.[39,56] The mechanism of detrusor overactivity might be related to the inhibitory effect of dopamine on micturition reflex. When pressure flow studies are done, a weak detrusor is found and is correlated with the stage of the disease. In addition, medications such as levodopa may also contribute to high resting urethral pressures. A long-standing question has been whether patients with Parkinson's disease or multisystem atrophy can safely undergo prostate surgery. No concerns were found with Parkinson's disease, but persistent urinary incontinence appeared in patients with multisystem atrophy.[42] Transurethral section of the prostate, therefore, can be done without risk of "de novo" urinary incontinence in Parkinson's disease.

Bladder dysfunction in multiple sclerosis is a consequence of spinal cord involvement and can be seen in acute relapse or in the more progressive forms. Again, the duration of the multiple sclerosis and the severity of pyramidal symptoms in the legs are predictive of bladder dysfunction.

The major neurourological problems are seen among patients who have a acute spinal cord injury.[8,9] Initially, all neurologic reflexes are absent, also known as the spinal shock stage. The bladder becomes atonic and there is no voluntary and supraspinal control of voiding.[12,14] Several months later, due to neuronal sprouting, spinal mediated reflexive voiding occurs and neurogenic detrusor overactivity occurs. This implies that there is disconnection from the pontine micturition center—voiding is determined largely by volume and reflex mechanisms in the detrusor. There is also a loss of sphincter detrusor activation. These contractions are highly inefficient, result in inadequate bladder emptying. The usual coordination between bladder and external urethral sphincter is absent and has been termed "detrusor sphincter dyssynergia." A Foley catheter is usually placed in patients who have urinary symptoms, which typically occur with lesions at or above the T-12 spinal level.

Patients with spinal cord lesions may have an acontractile detrusor, but in the vast majority, a detrusor sphincter dyssynergia or neurogenic detrusor overactivity occurs.[43] Anal pin sensation indicates intact fibers of the sensory spinothalamic tract in the spinal cord, and its preservation might be indicative of not only functional ambulation but also recovery of bladder function. Preservation of perianal pin sensation and bulbocavernous reflex is associated with higher chance of return of detrusor function within one year of injury, and many of those patients are able to urinate without assisted methods. In one recent study, 11 of 17 patients with preserved pin prick in the sacral area voided spontaneously despite presence of detrusor areflexia and detrusor hyperreflexia with more specific testing.[50]

Spinal cord lesions that produce bladder dysfunction are usually of three types: above spinal segment T6, below T6, or cauda equina. Lesions above T6 result in smooth sphincter dyssynergia, and lesions below T6 result in detrusor overactivity. A dyssynergic bladder causes poor bladder emptying and high detrusor pressure. Spinal cord lesions that are at the thoracolumbar level are usually associated with an acute detrusor areflexia. This has been seen as part of a "spinal shock." The bladder does not contract, and its improvement usually parallels the recovery of skeletal muscle reflexes. Usually bladder contractions will recommence in two months.[48] These patients have urinary incontinence and uninhibited contraction. Sacral lesions result in a contractile bladder; however, this areflexia is also associated with poor bladder compliance, resulting in progressive increase in intravesicular pressure with minimal filling. The external sphincter is not affected by sacral lesions, because the pelvic nerve innervation to the bladder occurs one segment higher than the pudendal nerve innervation of the sphincter. Bladder overdistension occurs with detrusor areflexia and intact sphincter function.

Bulbocavernosus (S2-S4), anal (S2-S5), and cremasteric reflexes (L1-L2) do differentiate levels of impairment.[34,52] The important rule is that any lesion of the sacral part of the spinal cord will lead to bladder dysfunction, except for patients with conus or cauda equina lesions that are limited to the S2-S4 segment.[29,35] These extreme caudal lesions may spare the bladder. Preserved sphincter tone but no voluntary contraction indicates a suprasacral lesion. Abnormal sphincter tone indicates a sacral lesion or peripheral (pudendal nerve) lesion.

In Practice

It is useful to integrate the neurological examination with urologic findings, and it may assist in helping to localize and anticipate the nature of the urologic problem. First, the abdomen is assessed for bladder enlargement (palpation and percussion). This may not be a simple assessment and may require a Doppler scan. Foley catheter placement reduces the chance of retention (if placed correctly). Failure to recognize an extended bladder may lead to renal failure and rapid rise in serum creatinine and amylase. An unrecognized full bladder can be a major cause of agitation in any neurologic patient and can be due to a simple obstruction.[2,15] In patients with spinal cord injury, the urinary bladder may go into spasm during catheter replacement, and the catheter balloon may easily be misplaced. A positive long catheter sign has been used to identify placement of Foley catheter in the urethra, but this remains subjective. X-ray of the pelvis with contrast may be helpful but is less useful than a simple CT scan of the pelvis.

The indications for catheterization are multifold, but in neurologic patients the benefits include more accurate urinary output measurement, management of acute urinary retention, and management of a neurogenic bladder.[46] Urinary catheterization improves patient comfort a great deal. The term "urinary catheter avoidance" is often invoked but difficult to achieve and would—at least in the early hospital days—require alternatives such as condom catheters, moisture-wicking incontinence pads, frequent catheterization, and frequent bladder scanning for monitoring bladder filling. However, urinary incontinence remains a dubious indication for placing an indwelling urethral catheter.

After urethral catheter placement, a closed system is attached, and such a system will reduce urinary tract infections. If urine is not obtained, pressure or tapping on the suprapubic region (Credé procedure[10]) may initiate flow; this procedure can be combined with irrigation of the catheter using 20 cc's of sterile saline, resulting in saline mixed with urine return.

The catheters are left in place and rarely changed. Timely removal of the urinary catheter in improving patients is encouraged. Usually, catheters can be removed after brain or spine surgery.[54] Once an indwelling catheter is placed and a prolonged catheterization is anticipated, a closed system should be maintained at all times. The drainage bay should be placed below the bladder, and the bag should be emptied when two-thirds full and before transport.

The risk of bacteriuria from catheter use increases daily and appears in approximately half of the patients who have been catheterized for more than a week.[19] Catheter-associated urinary tract infections are typically diagnosed with bacteriuria more than 100 colony forming (CFU) per ml, but often a positive urine culture is found in the absence of symptoms. Foley catheters are not currently coated. Some urinary catheters have silver impregnation, but there is no evidence that any of these catheters have reduced urinary tract infections, nor is there evidence that these catheters have increased antimicrobial resistance. Irrigation of the bladder is only performed if there is an obstruction. Routine sterile saline irrigation does not prevent urinary tract infection, not even when it includes antimicrobial irrigation. Trials using neomycin/polymyxin without irrigant did not reduce the incidence of urinary tract infections but did increase more resistant organisms.[31,41,44]

Intermittent catheterization is a long-term management procedure and effective and safe for bladder emptying by patient or caregiver (usually four times/day).[37] Urethral structures, although often mentioned, are not more common in patients with intermittent catheterization than in patients with indwelling catheters. Approximately 50% will at some point develop positive urine cultures, but most remain asymptomatic.

The treatment of neurogenic bladder typically involves antimuscarinic drugs[11] and avoidance of drug-induced urinary retention.[53] Antimuscarinic medication inhibits acetylcholine and muscarinic receptors and therefore improves both frequency and incontinence simply by relaxing the detrusor muscle. α-adrenergic receptors are in the proximal urethra, prostate, and bladder neck; therefore, blocking could help voiding and treat sphincter dyssynergia. The use of α-blockers is contraindicated in patients who have symptomatic hypotension. It is therefore not a good choice in patients with high-level spinal cord injuries, because their systolic blood pressures are mostly low—in the 100 mm Hg range.

Management of bladder also includes the management of infections and asymptomatic bacteriuria. Generally antibiotics are only prescribed if patients become symptomatic simply to avoid drug resistance associated with the use of prophylactic antibiotics. Prophylactic antibiotics are associated with reduction of incidence of asymptomatic bacteriuria, but they increase antibiotic resistance and do not prevent symptomatic infections. Moreover, recurrent upper urinary tract infections may indicate high bladder pressure or bladder stones that may need to be evaluated. Finally, in the evaluation of urinary retention, neurologic causes should be distinguished from nonneurologic causes (Table 9.2).[55] Any evaluation with bladder dysfunction involves evaluation for a urinary infection. Any patient with hematuria, renal impairment, recurrent urinary tract infections, or pain, likely associated with urinary tract, should be evaluated by a urologist.

Generally there is a consensus that conservative management to treat neurogenic detrusor overactivity and poor bladder emptying involves a combination of antimuscarinics and clean intermittent self-catheterization.[1,25,57] Intravesical capsaicin may be helpful.[20] Antimuscarinics remain the mainstay of treatment, and tolterodine 4 mg b.i.d. or botulism toxin is an effective treatment.[18,28,32,47] Botulinum toxin inhibits acetylcholine release at the neuromuscular junction and therefore relaxes spastic or overactive muscle. Its benefits have been seen up to 12 months after injection. A multicenter trial with patients assigned 200–300 units of Botox found significant improvement not only in urinary continence and

Table 9.2 **Causes of Urinary Retention**

Neurological Causes
• Detrusor external sphincter dyssynergia (e.g., due to myelopathy)
• Detrusor underactivity: loss of voluntary voiding (lesion of conus medullaris or spinal roots, multiple system atrophy, pure autonomic failure, radical pelvic surgery)
• Meningitis retention syndrome
Nonneurological Causes
• Primary disorder of urethral sphincter relaxation (Fowler's syndrome)
• Dysfunctional voiding (behavioral)
• Medications: anticholinergics, opiates
• Primary detrusor muscle failure

Modified from reference 34.

> **BY THE WAY**
> - Indwelling Foley catheters should not be replaced routinely
> - Bladder irrigation should be avoided unless to alleviate obstruction temporarily
> - Antimicrobial coated catheters do not reduce catheter-associated urinary tract infections
> - Breaks in closed drainage systems should lead to replacement

> **BLADDER DYSFUNCTION BY THE NUMBERS**
> - ~70% of urinary tract infections are preventable
> - ~50% of postoperative indwelling catheters may not be needed
> - ~50% of patients with neurogenic bladder can be treated
> - ~30% of all hospitalized patients suffer from urinary incontinence
> - ~25% of patients will receive an indwelling urinary catheter
> - ~5% daily increase of risk of bacteruria with catheter use

urodynamic parameters but also in quality of life. Combinations of antimuscarinics are also commonly used (trospium chloride 20 mg t.i.d. added to oxybutynin 5 mg t.i.d.).[11]

Surgical options are available, and sacral anterior root stimulation has been effective.[40] Sacral neuromodulation with implant has been considered early in spinal cord injury with the emergence of detrusor overactivity and, when tested, revealed absence of developing neurogenic detrusor overactivity or urinary incontinence when used early.[51]

Putting It All Together

- Bladder signals to the pontine micturition center occur with approximately 400 cc filling
- Parasympathetic output results in detrusor contraction and external sphincter control
- Urinary continence requires the ability to suppress detrusor contractibility
- Sympathetic output has a major role in urine storage via the pudendal nerve
- Acute urinary retention is an emergency but difficult to recognize after acute brain injury

- Urinary incontinence can be a disabling consequence of acute neurologic disease
- Treatment of neurogenic bladder involves antimuscarinic drugs or botulinum toxin

References

1. Abrams P, Agarwal M, Drake M, et al. A proposed guideline for the urological management of patients with spinal cord injury. *BJU Int* 2008;101:989–994.
2. Achong DM. Bladder outlet obstruction secondary to obstructed Foley catheter discovered on PET/CT. *Clin Nucl Med* 2010;35:341–342.
3. Andersson KE, Arner A. Urinary bladder contraction and relaxation: physiology and pathophysiology. *Physiol Rev* 2004;84:935–986.
4. Bacsu CD, Chan L, Tse V. Diagnosing detrusor sphincter dyssynergia in the neurological patient. *BJU Int* 2012;109 Suppl 3:31–34.
5. Benarroch EE. Neural control of the bladder: recent advances and neurologic implications. *Neurology* 2010;75:1839–1846.
6. Birder L, de Groat W, Mills I, Morrison J, Thor K, Drake M. Neural control of the lower urinary tract: peripheral and spinal mechanisms. *Neurourol Urodyn* 2010;29:128–139.
7. Blok BF, Willemsen AT, Holstege G. A PET study on brain control of micturition in humans. *Brain* 1997;120(Pt 1):111–121.
8. Burns AS, Rivas DA, Ditunno JF. The management of neurogenic bladder and sexual dysfunction after spinal cord injury. *Spine* 2001;26:S129–S136.
9. Cameron AP, Wallner LP, Forchheimer MB, et al. Medical and psychosocial complications associated with method of bladder management after traumatic spinal cord injury. *Arch Phys Med Rehabil* 2011;92:449–456.
10. Chang SM, Hou CL, Dong DQ, Zhang H. Urologic status of 74 spinal cord injury patients from the 1976 Tangshan earthquake, and managed for over 20 years using the Credé maneuver. *Spinal Cord* 2000;38:552–554.
11. Chapple CR, Khullar V, Gabriel Z, et al. The effects of antimuscarinic treatments in overactive bladder: an update of a systematic review and meta-analysis. *Eur Urol* 2008;54:543–562.
12. De Groat WC, Kawatani M, Hisamitsu T, Cheng CL, Ma CP, Thor K, Steers W, et al. Mechanisms underlying the recovery of urinary bladder function following spinal cord injury. *J Auton Nerv Syst* 1990;30 Suppl:S71–77.
13. De Groat WC, Yoshimura N. Pharmacology of the lower urinary tract. *Annu Rev Pharmacol Toxicol* 2001;41:691–721.
14. De Groat WC, Yoshimura N. Plasticity in reflex pathways to the lower urinary tract following spinal cord injury. *Exp Neurol* 2012;235:123–132.
15. De Luca GC, Wijdicks EFM. Images in clinical medicine. Agitation associated with acute bladder obstruction. *N Engl J Med* 2010;363:1656.
16. Drake MJ, Fowler CJ, Griffiths D, Mayer E, Paton JF, Birder L. Neural control of the lower urinary and gastrointestinal tracts: supraspinal CNS mechanisms. *Neurourol Urodyn* 2010;29:42–48.
17. Dumoulin C, Korner-Bitensky N, Tannenbaum C. Urinary incontinence after stroke: identification, assessment, and intervention by rehabilitation professionals in Canada. *Stroke* 2007;38:2745–2751.
18. Dykstra DD, Sidi AA, Scott AB, Pagel JM, Goldish GD. Effects of botulinum A toxin on detrusor-sphincter dyssynergia in spinal cord injury patients. *J Urol* 1988;139:919–922.
19. Esclarín De Ruz A, García Leoni E, Herruzo Cabrera R. Epidemiology and risk factors for urinary tract infection in patients with spinal cord injury. *J Urol* 2000;164:1285–1289.

20. Fowler CJ, Beck RO, Gerrard S, Betts CD, Fowler CG. Intravesical capsaicin for treatment of detrusor hyperreflexia. *J Neurol Neurosurg Psychiatry* 1994;57:169–173.
21. Fowler CJ, Dalton C, Panicker JN. Review of neurologic diseases for the urologist. *Urol Clin North Am* 2010;37:517–526.
22. Fowler CJ, Griffiths D, de Groat WC. The neural control of micturition. *Nat Rev Neurosci* 2008;9:453–466.
23. Fowler CJ, Griffiths DJ. A decade of functional brain imaging applied to bladder control. *Neurourol Urodyn* 2010;29:49–55.
24. Fowler CJ. Investigation of the neurogenic bladder. *J Neurol Neurosurg Psychiatry* 1996;60:6–13.
25. Fowler CJ. Systematic review of therapy for neurogenic detrusor overactivity. *Can Urol Assoc J* 2011;5:S146–S148.
26. Hansen RB, Biering-Sørensen F, Kristensen JK. Bladder emptying over a period of 10–45 years after a traumatic spinal cord injury. *Spinal Cord* 2004;42:631–637.
27. Holstege G. The emotional motor system and micturition control. *Neurourol Urodyn* 2010;29:119–127.
28. Kalsi V, Gonzales G, Popat R, et al. Botulinum injections for the treatment of bladder symptoms of multiple sclerosis. *Ann Neurol* 2007;62:452–457.
29. Kaplan SA, Chancellor MB, Blaivas JG. Bladder and sphincter behavior in patients with spinal cord lesions. *J Urol* 1991;146:113–117.
30. Kavia RB, Dasgupta R, Fowler CJ. Functional imaging and the central control of the bladder. *J Comp Neurol* 2005 5;493:27–32.
31. Niël-Weise BS, van den Broek PJ. Antibiotic policies for short-term catheter bladder drainage in adults. *Cochrane Database Syst Rev* 2005;3:CD005428.
32. Norlén L, Sundin T. Alpha-adrenolytic treatment in patients with autonomous bladders. *Acta Pharmacol Toxicol* (Copenh) 1978;43 Suppl 2:31–34.
33. Offermans MP, Du Moulin MF, Hamers JP, Dassen T, Halfens RJ. Prevalence of urinary incontinence and associated risk factors in nursing home residents: a systematic review. *Neurourol Urodyn* 2009;28:288–294.
34. Panicker JN, De Sèze M, Fowler CJ. Neurogenic lower urinary tract dysfunction. *Handb Clin Neurol*. 2013;110:209–220.
35. Pannek J, Stöhrer M, Blok B, et al. *Guidelines on Neurogenic Lower Urinary Tract Dysfunction*. European Association of Neurology. 2011. Available at www.uroweb.org
36. Patel M, Coshall C, Rudd AG, Wolfe CD. Natural history and effects on 2-year outcomes of urinary incontinence after stroke. *Stroke* 2001;32:122–127.
37. Perkash I, Giroux J. Clean intermittent catheterization in spinal cord injury patients: a followup study. *J Urol* 1993;149:1068–1071.
38. Pettersen R, Wyller TB. Prognostic significance of micturition disturbances after acute stroke. *J Am Geriatr Soc* 2006;54:1878–1884.
39. Ragab MM, Mohammed ES. Idiopathic Parkinson's disease patients at the urologic clinic. *Neurourol Urodyn* 2011;30:1258–1261.
40. Reynard JM, Vass J, Sullivan ME, Mamas M. Sphincterotomy and the treatment of detrusor-sphincter dyssynergia: current status, future prospects. *Spinal Cord* 2003;41:1–11.
41. Riley DK, Classen DC, Stevens LE, Burke JP. A large randomized clinical trial of a silver-impregnated urinary catheter: lack of efficacy and staphylococcal superinfection. *Is J Med* 1995;98:349–356.
42. Roth B, Studer UE, Fowler CJ, Kessler TM. Benign prostatic obstruction and Parkinson's disease—should transurethral resection of the prostate be avoided? *J Urol* 2009;181:2209–2213.
43. Sahai A, Cortes E, Seth J, et al. Neurogenic detrusor overactivity in patients with spinal cord injury: evaluation and management. *Curr Urol Rep* 2011;12:404–412.
44. Saint S, Elmore JG, Sullivan SD, Emerson SS, Koepsell TD. The efficacy of silver alloy-coated urinary catheters in preventing urinary tract infection: a meta-analysis. *Is J Med* 1998;105:236–241.

45. Saint S, Wiese J, Amory JK, et al. Are physicians aware of which of their patients have indwelling urinary catheters? *Is J Med* 2000;109:476–480.
46. Schumm K, Lam TB. Types of urethral catheters for management of short-term voiding problems in hospitalized adults: a short version Cochrane review. *Neurourol Urodyn* 2008;27:738–746.
47. Schurch B, de Sèze M, Denys P, et al. Botulinum toxin type A is a safe and effective treatment for neurogenic urinary incontinence: results of a single treatment, randomized, placebo controlled 6-month study. *J Urol* 2005;174:196–200.
48. Schurch B, Schmid DM, Karsenty G, Reitz A. Can neurologic examination predict type of detrusor sphincter-dyssynergia in patients with spinal cord injury? *Urology* 2005;65:243–246.
49. Seki S, Igawa Y, Kaidoh K, et al. Role of dopamine D1 and D2 receptors in the micturition reflex in conscious rats. *Neurourol Urodyn* 2001;20:105–113.
50. Shenot PJ, Rivas DA, Watanabe T, Chancellor MB. Early predictors of bladder recovery and urodynamics after spinal cord injury. *Neurourol Urodyn* 1998;17:25–29.
51. Sievert KD, Amend B, Gakis G, et al. Early sacral neuromodulation prevents urinary incontinence after complete spinal cord injury. *Ann Neurol* 2010;67:74–84.
52. Smith MD, Seth JH, Fowler CJ, Miller RF, Panicker JN. Urinary retention for the neurologist. *Pract Neurol*. 2013;13:288–291.
53. Verhamme KM, Sturkenboom MC, Stricker BH, Bosch R. Drug-induced urinary retention: incidence, management and prevention. *Drug Saf* 2008;31:373–388.
54. Wald HL, Ma A, Bratzler DW, Kramer AM. Indwelling urinary catheter use in the postoperative period: analysis of the national surgical infection prevention project data. *Arch Surg* 2008;143:551–557.
55. Watanabe T, Rivas DA, Chancellor MB. Urodynamics of spinal cord injury. *Urol Clin North Am* 1996;23:459–473.
56. Winge K, Nielsen KK. Bladder dysfunction in advanced Parkinson's disease. *Neurourol Urodyn* 2012;31:1279–1283.
57. Wyndaele JJ, Madersbacher H, Kovindha A. Conservative treatment of the neuropathic bladder in spinal cord injured patients. *Spinal Cord* 2001;39:294–300.

10

Troubleshooting: Localization Pearls

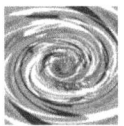

This book on recognizing acute injury to the central nervous system and its consequences assumes readers are able to examine such patients. Understanding the clinical consequences of acute neurologic disease—and how it changes neurologic examination—requires a process of neurological localization. Determining what underlies the acute presentation of certain neurologic conditions involves interpretation of neurologic findings, interpretation of neuroimaging, and interpretation of certain laboratory abnormalities. Only by systematically going through the motions can we achieve that. But there is something about it that causes many physicians to twist themselves into knots. This chapter shows how to troubleshoot.

The neurologic examination in acutely ill neurologic patients is markedly different from a neurologic examination in the office. In patients with a new brain lesion, the examination—apart from identifying focal signs—centers on brainstem reflexes, eye movement abnormalities, motor response to noxious stimuli, and patterns of weakness. In patients with a new spinal cord lesion, the examination proceeds first with identification of long tract signs and level of involvement using motor and sensory tests. In patients with acute muscle weakness, the response of tendon stretch reflexes and examination of neck muscles and jaw strength may be most revealing. In this chapter, we will review the basic necessities and neurologic skills of an examination in a patient with an acute neurologic disease. This mainly involves acute lesions of the brain, but because acute neurologic conditions could incidentally involve the spinal cord or result from acute neuromuscular disease, examination of these conditions is included (see other volume chapters for more details on acute neuromuscular conditions). Over many years, certain patterns have become apparent.

Principles

The practice of clinical localization must remain the major component of the practice of acute and emergency neurology. It requires a full knowledge of neurologic tests and cannot be truncated in an oversimplified scale or score. Many scores in use (NIHSS, ABCD2, GCS) provide minimal information and trivialize the importance of a good neurologic examination. Some are more detailed (e.g., FOUR score),[1] but none can (or should) replace a complete and individualized examination.

Though it would be ideal to always be able to predict precisely where the lesion is before we obtain neuroimaging, this would, for most of us, seem inconceivable. More often neuroimaging shows a lesion and physicians have to decide that what they see on the image matches what they find on examination. Physicians should not only understand the underlying anatomy but also how its interruption could account for the presentation and, in particular, how it may vary.[1-5] The proper way to do all that is presented here in the following sections.

FUNDAMENTALS OF LESION LOCALIZATION USING CLINICAL EXAMINATION

Perhaps not the most apt characterization, but, the brain can be artificially divided into sections: the hemispheres with their separate lobes, the brainstem, and the cerebellum. Each lesion will produce a combination of symptoms explained by the combination of the involved structures. These are summarized in Tables 10.1–10.3. It is necessary to point out that usually small lesions in the brainstem can produce major findings due to the compactness of the structures involved. In the cerebral hemispheres, large lesions can still be clinically silent, particularly in the right frontal lobe, and only some enlargement or mass effect impinging on other structures could result in noticeable symptomatology. Cerebral hemispheric lesions usually present themselves with disturbances in task switching, reasoning, perception, and memory, but also in weakness or, eventually, an abnormal level of consciousness. Lesions in the brainstem characteristically produce a cranial nerve deficit with or without hemiparesis.

Table 10.1 **Cerebral Hemispheres**

Frontal	
Right	May be silent
Left	Mood changes, abulia, poor execution
Temporal	
Right	Music-melody perception, Prosopagnosia
Left	Wernicke aphasia, apathy
Parietal	
Right	Neglect
Left	Poor calculation, poor 3D orientation
Occipital	
Right	Hemianopia
Left	Alexia without agraphia
	Abnormal color naming

Table 10.2 **Brainstem Lesions with Specific Localizations**

Mesencephalon	
Unilateral ventral	• Ipsilateral cranial nerve III (exiting fascicles of the cranial nerve III) • Contralateral hemiplegia (corticospinal)
Unilateral dorsal	• Ipsilateral cranial nerve III (nucleus) • Contralateral tremor or chorea (red nucleus)
Dorsal	• No upward gaze (colliculi) • Light-near dissociation (pupil fibers) • Lid retraction (posterior commissure levator fibers)
Ventral	• Abnormal consciousness (reticular formation) • Vertical gaze palsy (colliculi) • Miosis (sympathetic nerve)
Pons	
Base (unilateral)	• Ipsilateral cranial nerve VI and VII (fascicles) • Contralateral hemiplegia (corticospinal) • Ataxic hemiparesis (corticopontocerebellar fibers)
Ventral	• Locked-in syndrome • Quadriparesis (corticospinal) • Dysarthria (corticobulbar) • Absent horizontal movements (bilateral cranial nerve VI)
Dorsal	• Cerebellar dysarthria and rubral ataxia (cerebellar connections) • Tremor (red nucleus) • Sensory loss (spinothalamus)
Lateral	• Ipsilateral ataxia (cerebellar connections) • Contralateral hemiparesis (corticospinal) • Contralateral hypesthesia (spinothalamus tract)
Medulla Oblongata	
Lateral	• Contralateral loss of pain, temperature in body (Spinothalamic tract) • Ipsilateral loss of pain, temperature in face (trigeminal nucleus) • Ipsilateral ataxia (cerebellar peduncle) • Ipsilateral pharyngeal paralysis (nucleus ambiguus)
Medial	• Ipsilateral cranial nerve XII (nucleus) • Contralateral hemiparesis (corticospinal)

Table 10.3 **Cerebellum Lesions**

Vermis	
Rostral	• Ataxia of gait
	• Hypotonia, nystagmus, dysarthria
Hemisphere	
	• Incoordination and dysmetria (dentate nucleus)
	• Dysarthria
	• Nystagmus

Next, it is crucial to realize that although everything that presents itself seems acute, presentation of structural lesions can be either acute (due to a hemorrhage or infarction) or rapidly progressive (due to edema formation, mass effect, or both). An intracranial hematoma extending into the ventricles with initial localized symptoms may rapidly progress to coma. Acute lesions will have to be explained by an acute infarct or hemorrhage and require knowledge of the vascular supply of the cerebral hemispheres, brainstem, and cerebellum.

Anterior circulation syndromes such as a carotid artery syndrome or middle cerebral artery syndrome present with motor weakness affecting the opposite side involving face, arm, and leg; hemisensory loss; conjugate gaze or preference of eye position often also head movement toward the side of the lesion. There is a Broca aphasia noted with an infarct in the dominant hemisphere or a more global aphasia when the infarct is more extensive. When there is an infarction in the nondominant hemisphere, attention, neglect, denial, apraxia, or impaired prosody are found with careful observation.

Posterior circulation syndromes are far more complex and frequently are due to a mid or distal basilar artery occlusion that presents itself with acute ophthalmologic findings, usually involving the third or sixth nerve, but may result in acute ophthalmoplegia and pupillary abnormalities. The most notoriously difficult-to-recognize clinical syndrome is due to thalamic infarctions involving the posterior communicating artery and its perimesencephalic segment. Posterior circulation syndromes may involve a single thalamoperforator (artery of Percheron) and may be present in 1/3 of patients causing bithalamic infarcts and rostral midbrain infarcts all from one artery.

If the lesion is localized in the posterior cerebral artery, only an acute hemianopia is present. If there is bilateral occipital involvement, the patient may deny or be unaware of blindness. Bilateral occipital or para-occipital infarctions may be associated with optic ataxia (inability to grab objects), disturbance of visual attention, and simultanagnosia (inability to see two objects at the same time—i.e., pen and glasses). This combination is also known as Bálint's syndrome.

FUNDAMENTALS OF NEUROOPHTHALMOLOGY IN ACUTE NEUROLOGY

Pupil size is determined by the tone of the pupillodilator muscles and pupilloconstrictor muscles. Pupils can vary from 1–9 mm depending on ambient light. The innervation of the pupil is shown in Figure 10.1. The parasympathetic tract is far better to localize with shorter fibers from the Edinger-Westphal nucleus that travel with the third nerve to enter the sphincter pupillae. The sympathetic pathway is more complicated and starts at the posterior nucleus of the hypothalamus and projects to the hypothalamospinal tract to the lateral tegmentum of the midbrain, pons and medulla oblongata. The sympathetic fibers synapse with neurons in the intermediate gray of the thoracic spine segments and then travel through postganglionic fibers.

Miosis typically localizes to a pontine lesion, where the tegmentum involvement damages the sympathetic pathways. The light reflex (through the parasympathetic pathways) must be present, but changes in the miotic pupils cannot

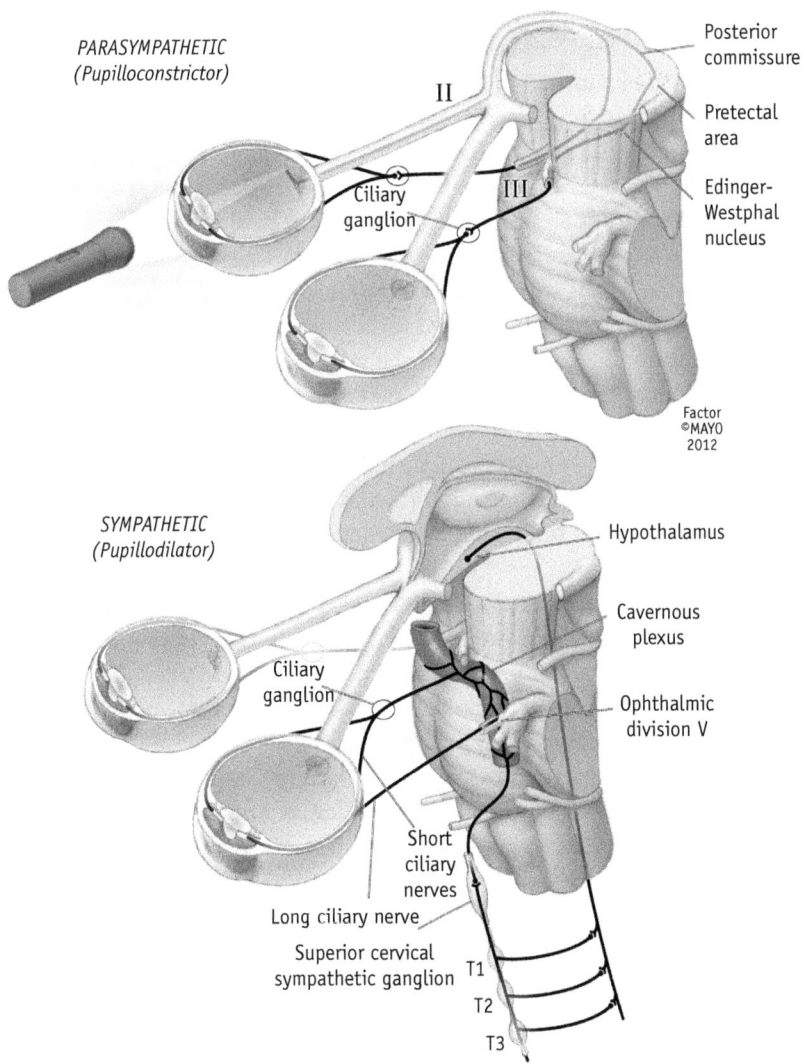

Figure 10.1 Parasympathetic and sympathetic inputs to the pupil.

be visibly observed (light reflex in pupils smaller than 2 mm cannot be reliably assessed with the naked eye).

Unilateral miosis (Horner's syndrome) may be due to involvement of the hypothalamus due to mass effect of a large hematoma, but it may also occur in a lesion without significant mass effect (ipsilateral to temporal lobe hematoma). It may also occur with lateral medulla oblongata lesions.

As expected, tectal lesions of the midbrain result in light-fixed pupils. When the midbrain lesion interrupts both sympathetic and parasympathetic tracts, the pupils are midway (5 mm) fixed and the first sign of more significant injury. Traditionally, it has been taught that pupil responses remain intact even in an acute metabolic derangement or intoxication. Actually, pupils may change and lose light response with a high intravenous dose of barbiturates, but not high doses of benzodiazepine or propofol. Intravenous drugs (i.e., atropine), locally applied drugs, or mists from bronchodilators occasionally surprise physicians as a cause for a dilated pupil.

In the examination of the comatose patient, attention to eye movements and eye position can be quite diagnostic. The eyes, when abnormal (movement, position, and pupils), provide crucial information. The reflex pathways are dorsally in the brainstem and thus abnormal eye reflexes may be a telltale sign of injury in the region where the reticular formation is located.

Our understanding of eye movements is as follows: brief, rapid, voluntary, conjugate horizontal movements are fired from the frontal lobe. Bundles from this eye field in the frontal lobe descend to the midbrain and cross at the location of the trochlear nerve to synapse with the paramedian pontine reticular formation and sixth nerve nucleus. Rapid voluntary vertical movements are fired from bilateral frontal and occipital eye fields synapsing at the junction of midbrain and thalamus, predominantly in the tegmentum, and connecting to oculomotor nuclei. Abnormal resting eye positions indicate lesions in the supranuclear pathways of conjugate eye movements.

After opening the eyelids, one should assess the eyes' position and whether they spontaneously move. Roving eye movements simply indicate a much lower likelihood of severe brain injury, and not only, as is typically taught, absence of brainstem injury. Completely immobile ("frozen") eyes indicate brainstem injury, a major toxin, or neuromuscular junction blockers.

Lateral conjugate deviation of the eyes toward the lesion indicates a destructive, mostly large frontotemporal parietal lesion. A horizontal conjugate deviation away from the lesion indicates a seizure (focal initially and often becoming generalized later). Sustained upward gaze is typical of a diffused hemispheric lesion, but the pathway is not known. Sustained downward gaze is due to thalamus hemorrhage or lesion in the dorsal midbrain (e.g., tumor or hydrocephalus).

The pons controls horizontal conjugate eye movement, with the abducens nucleus as the most important controller. The abducens projects up to the contralateral oculomotor nucleus through the medial longitudinal fasciculus. Inputs come from vestibular nuclei and frontal eye fields. Skew deviation is looked at next. This is caused by interruption of pathways at the lateral medulla oblangata (rostral), pons (lower part), vestibular nucleus, or cerebellum.

Skew deviation in the resting position is indicative of a primary brainstem lesion, possibly in the region of the interstitial nucleus of Cajal. The higher eye is often at a site similar to that of the midbrain or pons lesion.

Brainstem lesions may interrupt the medial longitudinal fasciculus and can be demonstrated with caloric stimulation. Caloric stimulation with ice water stimulates horizontal canals with the head elevated 30° and produces a tonic deviation toward the ear, but it may bring out an adduction paralysis (internuclear ophthalmoplegia). Skew deviation may be associated with diplopia and indicates an internuclear lesion. It is a result of abnormalities in fibers ascending vertically from vestibular nuclei with the medial longitudinal fasciculus.

FUNDAMENTALS OF FUNCTIONAL ANATOMY IN COMA EXAMINATION

The neuroanatomical correlates of arousal and awareness have been discussed in Chapter 4. The implication of this organizational structure is that coma is caused by an interruption in any of these circuits. Clinicopathologic correlations have been published, and there is an agreement among clinicians that certain locations can cause unconsciousness and combinations of these locations can cause permanent unconsciousness.

The three honored questions that need to be asked in order to elucidate the cause of coma are:

1. Is it a destructive structural lesion or is it due to a global acute physiologic derangement of brain function?
2. Is the structural lesion hemispheric or in the brainstem?
3. Is the lesion inside the brainstem or due to displacement of the brainstem?

Knowing these elements, a more specific localization can be made, and useful templates are shown in Table 10.4. The clinical signs of brainstem displacement likely reflect the change in geometry. What is noted clinically is a summation of damage of each involved structure. Brainstem displacement and compression are often maximal at the onset of an acute, rapidly expanding mass lesion. In more slowly expanding lesions (e.g., hemispheric ischemic edema), clinical signs are due to more compression effects and not necessarily more shift.

Bihemispheric cortical injury should be diffuse to cause coma. Destructive damage involving the entire cortical mantle can occur with anoxic-ischemic injury, although the parieto-occipital regions are most severely affected. The white matter core can be damaged mostly from acute demyelinating disorders or from acute

Table 10.4 **The Comatose Patient**

Location	Clinical Pointers
Bihemispheric	• Spontaneous eye movements (roving, dipping, ping-pong) • Upward or downward eye deviation • Intact oculovestibular responses • Intact brainstem reflexes • Variable motor responses • Myoclonus status epilepticus
Intrinsic brainstem	• Skew deviation • Internuclear ophthalmoplegia • Downbeat nystagmus • Miosis • Variable pupil or corneal reflexes (may both be absent) • Absent oculocephalic or oculovestibular responses • Extensor or flexion motor responses
Brainstem displacement (from hemispheric or cerebellar mass)	• Anisocoria or unilateral fixed wide pupil (lateral displacement from hemispheric mass) • Midposition fixed pupils (downward central displacement from hemispheric mass) • Absent corneal reflexes and intact pupil reflexes (displacement from cerebellar mass) • Extensor or flexion motor responses

hydrocephalus and this will interrupt the thalamocortical circuits. The thalamus can be preferentially affected, usually due to ischemic injury from both arterial and venous occlusions, but in most instances, function is impaired due to compression from a new mass. Thalamic injury leads to a de-efferentiated (to the cortex) and de-afferentiated (from the reticular formation) state. Involvement of the dorsal parts of the mesencephalon, pons, and pontomedullary border interrupts wakefulness by disconnecting from the thalamus, hypothalamus, and cortex.

The hemispheres in comatose patients can only be examined by gross assessment of responses to sound, touch, and noxious stimuli. The thalamus and upper brainstem may produce more localizable signs. Therefore, before detailed features of the neurologic examination are described, it is useful to revisit the important reflex circuits.

A lesion in the tectum or pretectum with involvement of the posterior commissure fixes the pupil to a light swung in front of the pupil. When the third nerve nucleus (Edinger-Westphal) is involved, the pupil fixes in midposition. Stretch or compression of the oculomotor nerve or compression of the midbrain oculomotor

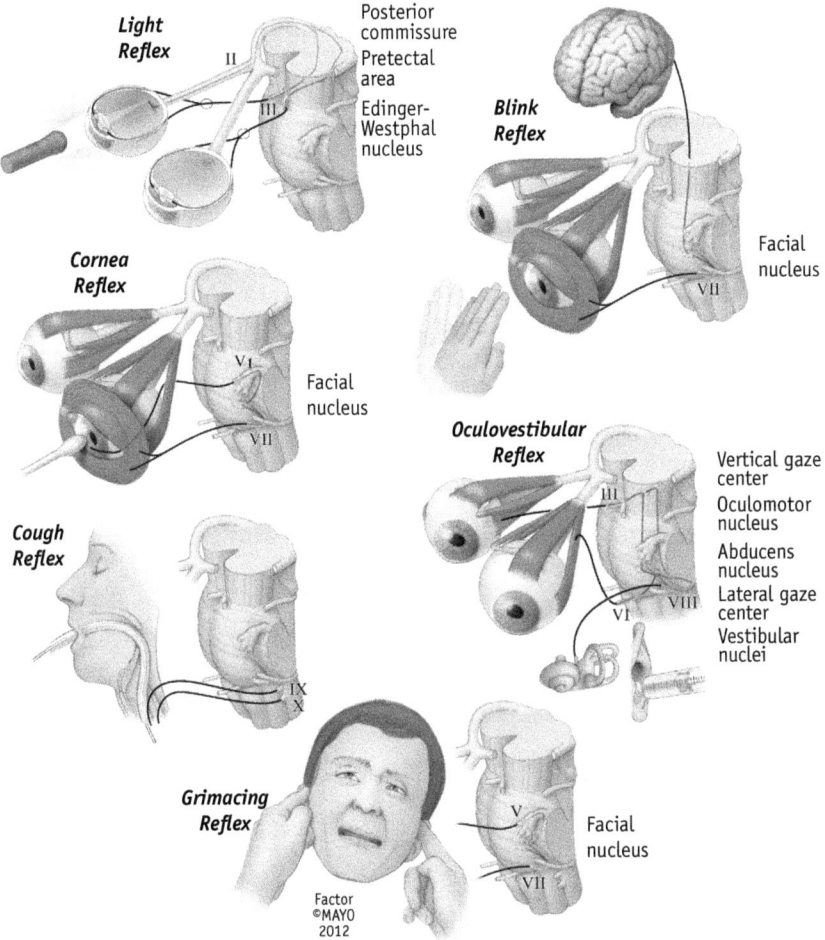

Figure 10.2 Brainstem reflexes in patients with abnormal consciousness. (From reference 1.)

complex results in a dilated pupil due to intact unopposed sympathetic pathway. Conversely, pinpoint pupils are seen in pontine lesions due to damage to descending sympathetic fibers, but the light reflex is intact.

The blink reflex arc is complex, depending on the stimulus (Figure 10.2). This stimulus is usually a rapid-hand approach (optic nerve is the afferent part) or sound (acoustic nerve is the afferent part). The afferent parts are the orbicularis oculi muscles innervated by the facial nerve. An intact visual system, including a functioning visual cortex, is needed to cause blinking after a visual stimulus. However, the acoustic arc is through the brainstem, and blinking after a loud sound does not need cortical input. This difference is useful when examining patients with severe hemispheric injury and intact brainstem function, such as in a persistent vegetative state. Visual tracking requires cortical input from the primary visual cortex and frontal eye field (Figure 10.2). Horizontal visual tracking is a coordinated response using the lateral gaze center or pontine paramedian reticular formation. It activates the oculomotor nucleus in the mesencephalon and the abducens nucleus in the pons. The ascending pathway from the lateral gaze center to the oculomotor center is known as the medial longitudinal fasciculus. Vertical visual tracking is coordinated through the vertical gaze center present in the periaqueductal gray matter of the mesencephalon. It projects to the oculomotor and trochlear nuclei.

The corneal reflex is elicited after touching the cornea. The ophthalmic (I) division of the trigeminal nerve (nasociliary branch) synapses with the motor division of the facial nerve that contracts the orbicularis oculi muscles. An oculovestibular reflex can be elicited in comatose patients. It does require detection of cold (ice) water by the semicircular canals, signaling through the eighth cranial nerve to the vestibular nuclei, and projecting to third, fourth, and sixth nuclei via the gaze centers. This results in a tonic movement of the eyes toward the cold stimulus (Figure 10.2). Internuclear ophthalmoplegia involves a lesion of the medial longitudinal fasciculus in the upper pons and can be documented with caloric testing. Its presence reveals a pontine lesion. The cough reflex is usually best elicited with tracheal suctioning. It consists of a pathway from the sensory laryngeal nerve to the efferent vagal nerve (Figure 10.2).

FUNDAMENTALS OF FUNCTIONAL ANATOMY IN ACUTE GENERALIZED WEAKNESS

The neurologic examination of the weak patient should include inspection of spontaneous movements (fasciculations, myokymia) and skin (erythema, purpura, ulcerations). Muscle weakness can be graded, but strength is often an approximation as a result of cooperation from the sick patient. Bilateral flaccid paralysis of the arms and legs or of the arms more than the legs may indicate an acute spinal cord lesion, certainly if the anal reflex is lost, body temperature is low, the skin is warm, and priapism and dysautonomia are present. Distal weakness is common in neuropathies, and proximal weakness is common in inflammatory polyneuropathies.

Neurologic examination may detect areflexia, atrophy causing prominence of the hand tendons and tibia (e.g., in polyneuropathy, amyotrophic lateral sclerosis), fatigability of upward gaze producing worsening ptosis, and weakness of the masseter muscle (myasthenia gravis). Quadriplegia or paraparesis may have its origin in the spinal cord. Hypotonia, failure to control bladder and bowel sphincters, areflexia, and a distinct sensory level to pinprick are found initially. Sensory loss may be suggested by failure of the patient to grimace or retract to a noxious stimulus, but careful evaluation of sensory level is not always reliable. The patient needs to display adequate attention for the physician to detect a possible thoracic level of pinprick analgesia.

Neurologic examination should localize the lesion in patients with acute paraplegia or tetraplegia. Sensory abnormalities localize in the vertical plane (cervical, lumbar, sacral) and, when combined with other long-tract signs, point to localization in the horizontal plane (extradural, intradural, or intramedullary). The sensory dermatomes are important for localization.

The degree of spinal cord involvement is graded to determine whether the lesion is complete or incomplete. It is complete when absence of both motor and sensory function below the lesion level is documented. The degree of weakness can be assessed by grading muscle strength on the grading scale of the British Medical Research Council. Although one may grade the weakness of all muscles for documentation and comparison over time, some muscles are localizing: arm abduction (C5), forearm extension (C5), forearm flexion (C5 and C6), knee extension (L3 and L4), foot and great toe dorsiflexion (L5), and plantar flexion (S1).

Assessing muscle tone is also important, although many patients have a flaccid paralysis due to so-called spinal shock—a poorly understood pathophysiologic phenomenon. Muscle tone, or the resistance a muscle has against passive movement of the joint, may distinguish between upper motor neuron disease and lower motor neuron disease. Upper motor neuron disease typically causes spasticity in which the flexors in the upper extremities and extensors to the lower extremities are more commonly involved. It is worthwhile to inspect the muscles for atrophy, which may indicate a long-standing process that has evolved into cord compression. Acute radiculopathy does not produce atrophy, but long-standing compression root lesions produce fasciculations and significant atrophy of the muscle bulk. Myoclonic twitching may occur and can be widespread in acute spinal cord injury.

All sensory modalities should be tested (pinprick, position, and vibration sense; light touch with a wisp of cotton; pressure touch; and temperature). Abnormal pinprick is usually interpreted as touch without identification of a sharp sting and is most valuable in localizing segments. When a tuning fork is unavailable to test vibration, at least position sense should be tested. Normally, movement of a few degrees in the position of the toe joints should be easily appreciated. In addition, tactile discrimination should be tested, and normally a 2- to 3-cm difference between two points should be appreciated. Normal function suggests intact posterior column tracts but also nerve root function.

Saddle anesthesia (S3-S5) is an indication of a conus medullaris lesion, which can be accurately delineated but may be missed with superficial examination in a supine patient. The sensory loss is often dissociated, with sparing of touch but loss of pinprick. Absence of dissociation suggests involvement of the cauda equina, not just the conus.

Sacral sparing of the sensory symptoms is an important sign because it implies a centrally located intramedullary lesion. The representation of the sacral fibers is very peripheral in the cord; thus, pinprick and temperature sensation may be spared in acute central cord lesions.

The presence of abnormal sensory findings of different modalities may further localize. Brown-Séquard syndrome is strongly indicative of extramedullary compression, and it may occur in patients with cancer and radiation myelopathy. Its clinical hallmark is loss of pain and temperature sensation opposite the lesion, with loss of position and vibration, and more prominent leg weakness, at the level of the lesion. The patient often is puzzled by numbness in one leg and weakness in the other. Brown-Séquard syndrome is rarely uniform in presentation, but marked unilateral leg weakness with a Babinski sign and lack of position recognition of the toe should point to acute extramedullary compression. The classic patterns of sensory loss in myelopathies are depicted in Figure 10.3.

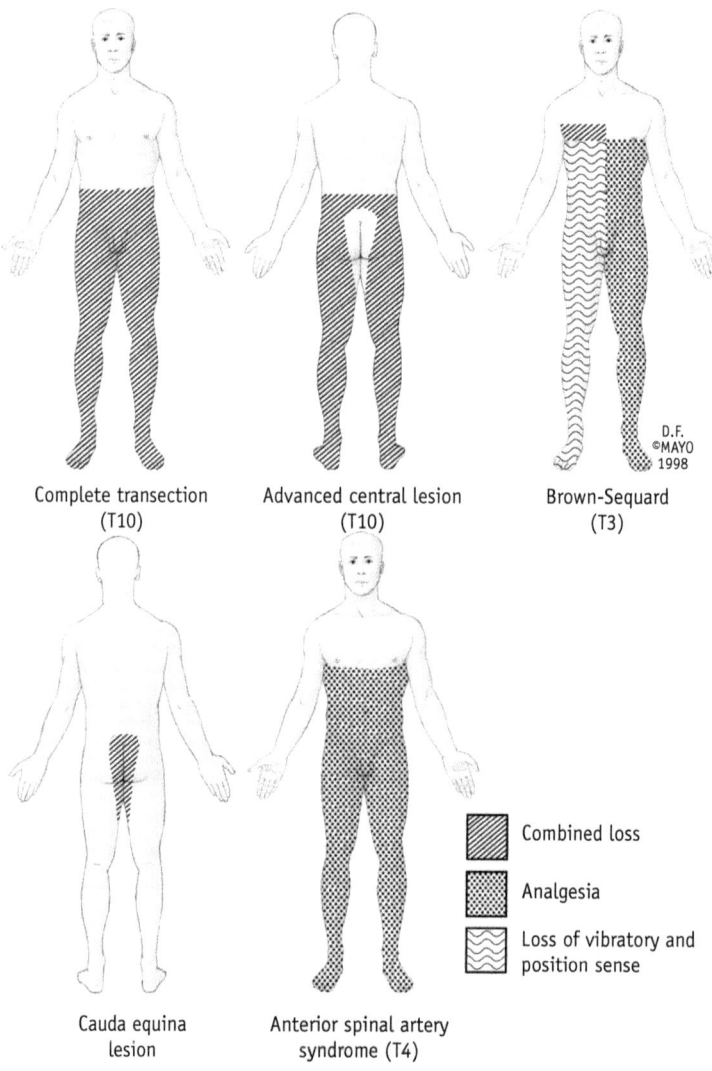

Figure 10.3 Localization of lesions in the spinal cord. (From Reference 2.)

In Practice

Now how would we go about localizing these findings? There are at least five major misjudgments in localization in acute neurology.

The first misjudgment is failure to localize abnormalities in the brainstem. Where clinicians get sidetracked is failure to appreciate the combination of abnormal cranial nerve findings with abnormal motor responses. A patient with abnormal pupils, anisocoria, and extensor posturing must have a lesion where the individual fibers are closely located in a small structure.

The second misjudgment is failure to localize the lesion in both hemispheres. Coma with bilateral abnormal motor responses and no eye findings localizes to both hemispheres. Often a CT scan may initially show findings in one hemisphere (evolving stroke or encephalitis), confusing the clinician, who has to return to the basic neurologic findings to conclude that more than one hemisphere is involved.

The third misjudgment is failure to localize in the cerebellum. Patients may have a gait instability that may not have been tested. Vomiting is more common than a patient volunteers and vertigo may not be mentioned if the patient is not asked. Dysarthria needs to be brought about by asking the patient to repeat a sentence (i.e., the child takes the bus to school every morning), and then poorly articulated speech will appear.

The fourth misjudgment is the failure to appreciate spinal cord injury, to identify a sensory level, and to narrow down the segments involved with motor weakness. Again, important pointers are nipple at level T4; umbilicus at level T10; and thumb, middle finger, and fifth digit innervated by C6, C7, and C8. The C4 and T2 dermatomes are continuous.

The fifth misjudgment is failure to clinically recognize deterioration of the patient. Deterioration in a patient with an acute brain injury is disease specific but predictable in many acute disorders. Examples are shown in Table 10.5. Serial CT scan also remains the most useful method of monitoring structural central nervous system lesions. Portable CT scan may even be more helpful, but there are no comparative studies yet. CT scan is able to document enlargement of ventricles, signs of mass effect with further displacement of the pineal gland and septum pellucidum, obliteration of basal cisterns and sulcal effacement, compression of the brainstem, and intraventricular extension of hemorrhage, among other signs of a changing lesion.

In many instances, neurologic deterioration is due to further displacement of brain tissue and eventually brainstem displacement. Lateral brain tissue shift distorts the thalamus and mesencephalon. These patients present with decline in consciousness (thalamus-mesencephalon). Unilateral fixed dilated (varying from 2- to 5-millimeter difference) pupil is seen early and can be followed by bilateral fixed pupils. The pontine reflexes remain intact. This course, however, can be mimicked by acute lesions in the thalamus that suddenly extend asymmetrically to the mesencephalon (e.g., thalamic hemorrhage). In patients with a gaze preference toward the

Table 10.5 **Causes of Clinical Deterioration in Selected Disorders**

Disorder	Causes of Clinical Deterioration	Clinical Signs of Deterioration
Aneurysmal subarachnoid hemorrhage	• Acute hydrocephalus • Delayed cerebral ischemia • Rebleeding • Expanding lobar hematoma • Seizures	• Decline in consciousness • Upward gaze palsy • Pinpoint pupils • Sudden loss of upper brainstem reflexes and transient apnea
Ganglionic or lobar hemorrhage	• Expanding volume • Rebleeding	• New aphasia or hemiparesis • Eye deviation • Decrease consciousness • Worsening hemiparesis
Cerebellar hematoma	• Compression of fourth ventricle and acute hydrocephalus • Displacement of pons	• Acute anisocoria or wide fixed pupil and extensor posturing • New acute hypertension • Pinpoint pupils and downward gaze
Hemispheric infarct	• Hemorrhagic conversion • Brain swelling	• Comatose and need for intubation • Sudden coma with extensor posturing and midposition pupils.
Traumatic brain injury	• New contusional lesions • Malignant cerebral edema • Extension of subdural or epidural hematoma	• Gradual decline in consciousness. • New onset cerebral ptosis • New fixed dilated pupil. • New decerebrate or decorticate responses.

expanding mass, the gaze may reverse due to thalamic compression. A lateral fixed gaze may occur. Further vertical displacement of the entire thalamus-mesencephalon pontine structure may occur, but only after the upper brainstem has been destroyed directly from compression. It may occur with bilateral thalamic compression from diffuse brain edema. Patients who lose all brainstem reflexes usually lose ponto-mesencephalic reflexes at onset and medulla oblangata function later. A common progression is appearance of flaccidity and no motor response with loss of ponto-mesencephalic reflexes and, finally, failure to trigger the ventilator, indicating brain death. The degree of involvement determines the reversibility of coma.

Lesions in the cerebellum may produce compression of the brainstem but more at the pontine level. Most notable is a predominance of pontine signs with possible bilateral miosis, loss of both corneal reflexes and oculocephalic reflexes. Frequent episodes of bradycardia with or without hypertension may occur (Cushing reflex). A mass located more centrally compresses the thalamus and mesencephalon in a vertical plane, causing fixed midposition (4–6 mm) pupils initially. Asymmetric compression of the mesencephalon with anisocoria and the larger pupil or an oval-shaped pupil at the site of the lesion may be seen. Motor responses vary from decorticate to extensor responses, with sometimes even variation throughout the day and no evidence of other signs of deterioration.

Coma can be reversible when the displacing mass is removed. Brainstem compression from a hemorrhage in the cerebellum or swollen infarct has the best chance of improvement, assuming the mass effect can be removed with suboccipital craniotomy. Removal of supratentorial hematomas can be very successful after the patient continues to deteriorate. Removal of a lobar hematoma with extension into the thalamus, however, is likely unsuccessful because the damage involves a key structure. Removal of mass effect will not lead to improvement of the patient if the thalamus is destroyed. In some patients, displacement or compression of the ventricular system can lead to an acute hydrocephalus, and a ventriculostomy can lead to marked improvement in level of consciousness. This scenario is seen in patients with cerebellar hemorrhage in which a rapid or gradual decline in consciousness could be partly due to obstruction and ventricular enlargement.

Putting It All Together

- Eye movement, pupil reflexes, and eye position are important localizing clues of acute brain injury
- Deterioration from both supratentorial and infratentorial masses can be predicted
- Neurologic examination should be interpreted together with acutely obtained neuroimaging
- Recognition of spinal cord injury requires recognition of sensory abnormalities together with long tract signs can localize in the spinal cord

References

1. Wijdicks EFM. *The Comatose Patient*, 2nd edition. New York, Oxford University Press, 2014.
2. Wijdicks EFM. *The Practice of Emergency and Critical Care Neurology*. New York, Oxford University Press, 2010.
3. Brazis PW, Masdeu JC, Biller J. *Localization in Clinical Neurology* 6th ed. Philadelphia, Lippincott Williams and Wilkins, 2011.
4. Ropper AH, Samuels MA., Klein JP. *Adams and Victor's Principles of Neurology*. 10th ed. New York, McGraw-Hill Medical, 2014.
5. Caplan LR, Van Gijn J. *Stroke syndromes* 3rd ed. New York, Cambridge University Press, 2012.

Index

Page numbers followed by 'f' refer to figures.

acetazolamide 33, 38
acetylcholine 93, 106
adrenaline (epinephrine) 78, 84, 87, 91
akinetic mutism 48, 52
α-adrenergic agonists. *See* clonidine;
    norepinephrine; phenylephrine
α-adrenergic receptors 78, 82, 84f, 125–6
amantadine 53
amiodarone 99–100
amlodipine 82
AMPA receptors 4
analgesics 26
    See also opioids
aneurysmal subarachnoid hemorrhage 35, 86, 96,
    99, 142
angiotensin receptor blockers 82
anoxic–ischemic injury 3–4, 47, 135
anterior cingulate cortex 45, 48, 108, 118
anterior circulation syndromes 132
antiarrhythmic drugs 99–100
antibiotics 37, 124
anticoagulants 37, 40
antidiuretic hormone (vasopressin) 84, 85, 87, 88, 97
antihypertensive drugs 81–83, 86–87
antimuscarinic drugs 124–25
anxiety 72
aortic aneurysm repair 40–41
aphasia 132
apnea
    brain death 74–75
    sleep 64, 65
apneustic breathing 64
apneustic center 61
apoptosis 4, 5f, 6, 7, 8
arrhythmias 84, 94, 95f, 96, 97, 99–101
arterial blood gases
    apnea test 74–75
    cerebral blood flow and 80
    in respiration 61–63, 62f, 66, 68, 72

ascending activating reticular system
    (ARAS) 45, 46
assist control ventilation 69f
ataxic respiration (Biot breathing) 64
atenolol 81
atomoxetine 54
atrial fibrillation 96, 99
atrial natriuretic peptide 96
atrioventricular (AV) node 92, 93
autonomic nervous system
    bladder function 118–20, 118f, 119f
    blood pressure 22, 78–79, 79f, 86–87
    cardiac function 92–94, 92f,
    gastrointestinal function 106, 107f, 108, 112
    pupil size 133, 133f
axonal injury 5–6
    demyelination 6–7, 8

bacterial overgrowth in the gut 109–10
Bainbridge reflex 96
barbiturates 25, 26, 134
baroreceptors 79, 96
Barrington's nucleus (pontine micturition center)
    117–18
basal energy expenditure (BEE) 110–11
β-adrenergic receptors 78, 84f, 93
β-blockers 82, 86, 86, 99, 100
Bezold–Jarisch reflex 96
bilevel positive airway pressure (BiPAP) 68
biomarkers of neuronal injury 11–12
Biot breathing 64
bladder 117–26
    anatomy and physiology 117–20, 118f, 119f
    neurological disorders 120–26
blink reflex 136, 137f
blood gases. *See* arterial blood gases
blood pressure 77–88
    hypertension 77, 80, 81–83, 85–86
    hypotension 12–13, 31, 77, 83–85, 87–88

blood pressure (*Cont.*)
  ICP and 20, 22, 25, 81
  physiology 78–81, 79f, 80f
blood-brain barrier 4, 6, 12
botulism toxin 124–25
bradycardia 83, 94, 96, 143
brain death 9, 74–75, 142
brain edema. *See* cerebral edema
brain natriuretic peptide 96
brainstem
  anoxic–ischemic injury 3
  blood pressure control 79
  breathing and 60–61, 60f, 64, 65
  consciousness and 44–45, 46, 48
  displacement 22, 135, 138, 141–43
  localization of injuries 35, 131, 134–35, 136, 138, 141
  raised ICP 17, 22
breathing 59–76
  assistance with 65, 67–74, 69f
  central causes of abnormal breathing 35, 63–65
  peripheral causes of abnormal breathing 66
  physiology 59–63, 61f
Brown-Séquard syndrome 140, 140f
buspirone 26

calcium channel blockers 82, 86
calcium ions 4
caloric stimulation 135, 136–37
carbon dioxide
  apnea test 74–75
  breathing 61–63, 62f, 68, 72
  cerebral blood volume and 19, 31, 81
cardiac function 91–101
  anatomy and physiology 92–97, 92f
  arrhythmias 82, 94, 95f, 96, 97, 99–101
  drugs affecting 82–85
  EKG abnormalities 98–99
  stress-induced cardiomyopathy 91, 94–95, 96, 97–98
cardiogenic shock 85, 87
carotid bodies 62, 96
caspases 4, 7
catecholamines. *See* dopamine; epinephrine; norepinephrine
catheterization, urinary 123
cauda equina lesions 120, 122, 139, 140f
central neurogenic hyperventilation 64
central sleep apnea 64, 65
cerebellum 3, 132, 141, 142, 143
cerebral blood flow
  blood pressure and 20, 79–81, 80f
  ICP and 20, 22, 40
  in infections 6–7
  neuronal function 81
cerebral blood volume 19, 25, 40
cerebral cortex
  anoxic–ischemic injury 3–4, 135
  bladder control 118, 121

breathing 60
cardiac function 96–97
consciousness/unconsciousness 45, 46, 47, 48–50
gastrointestinal control 108
spreading depression 11
cerebral edema 6, 7–9, 12, 80
cerebral perfusion pressure (CPP) 20, 22, 24–25, 35, 80
cerebrospinal fluid (CSF) 29–41
  in aortic aneurysm repair 40–41
  bloody 24
  hydrocephalus 19, 29, 34–38, 36f, 40, 143
  ICP and 18, 19, 34, 35
  leaks 38–40
  physiology 30–34, 30f, 32f, 33f, 62
chemoreceptors 62, 96
Cheyne-Stokes breathing 64, 65
children 6
cholecystokinin 106, 108
choroid plexus 31, 32f, 33
cisapride 114
clinical examination 52, 129–43, 137f
clonidine 26, 82, 86, 96
coagulation 7
  anticoagulants 37, 40
colonic motility 105, 106, 108–9, 113–14
coma 43–54
  examination 52–53, 134, 135–37, 137f, 138, 141–42
  management 46, 53–54
  neuroanatomy and neurophysiology of consciousness 44–48, 45f
  neuroimaging 43, 48–51, 49f, 50f, 52
  scales 130
communication with patients in MCS 50–51
computed tomography (CT) 141
  cerebral edema 12
  CSF leaks 38
  hydrocephalus 35
consciousness 43
  declining 35, 141–42
  neuroanatomy/neurophysiology 44–47, 45f
  See also unconsciousness
continuous positive airway pressure (CPAP) 69f, 70, 72
contraction band necrosis 94f, 96
contusions 6
corneal reflex 136, 137f
cortex. *See* cerebral cortex
corticosteroids 34, 87
cough reflex 137, 137f
CPAP (continuous positive airway pressure) 69f, 70, 72
CPP (cerebral perfusion pressure) 20, 22, 24–25, 35, 80
CSF. *See* cerebrospinal fluid
CT. *See* computed tomography
cuneus 48, 50
Cushing reflex 143

Cushing ulcers 112
cytotoxic edema 6, 9

death. *See* brain death
deep brain stimulation 54
default mode network 49–50, 49f
dehydration 83, 87
delirium 51–52
demyelination 6–7, 8
deterioration of a patient 12–13, 81, 141–42
detrusor areflexia 122
detrusor hyperreflexia (overactive bladder) 120, 121, 122, 124
detrusor sphincter dyssynergia 120, 121, 122
dexmedetomidine 26, 86
diaphragm 63, 66, 68
dietary supplements 110
dihydroergotamine 25
diltiazem 82, 100
disconnection syndrome 48
diuretics
  antihypertensive 81
  osmotic 20, 22–23, 23f, 25, 31
dobutamine 84, 85, 87
domperidone 114
dopamine
  blood pressure 78, 83, 85, 87
  wakefulness 46, 54
dorsal respiratory group (DRG) 61
dural sinus pressure 34
dyspnea 60, 63–66
  management 65, 67–74, 69f

echocardiography 97
electrocardiography (EKG) 98–99
electroencephalography (EEG) 9, 10, 11, 26, 51
electrolytes, in CSF 31
endoscopy 113
energy metabolism 1, 11, 14
enteral nutrition 109, 111
epilepsy 7, 96
  See also seizures
epinephrine 78, 84, 87, 91
erythromycin 109, 114
esmolol 86, 100
excitotoxicity 4, 5, 7
eye examinations 35, 132–35, 137f
  in comatose patients 52, 134, 136, 141–42
  gaze abnormalities 35, 52, 134–35, 136, 142

face masks 67, 68
feeding 109–11
fentanyl 26, 65
fluid resuscitation 83, 87
fluoxetine 54
Forrest grade 113
frontal lobe 49, 118, 120, 130, 134
functional magnetic resonance imaging (fMRI) 43, 48–51, 49f, 50f, 53

gamma-aminobutyric acid (GABA) 46
gastrointestinal system 105–15
  anatomy and physiology 106–9, 107f
  hemorrhage 112–13, 114
  motility 105, 106, 108–9, 113–14
  nutrition 109–11
  stress ulcers 108, 112–13
gastroparesis 108–9, 113
gastrosotomy 111
gaze abnormalities 35, 52, 134–35, 136, 142
ghrelin 108
glial cells 12
global diffuse ischemia (hypoxic–ischemic injury) 3, 35
glucagon-like peptide (GLP-1) 108
glucose 31, 81
  hypoglycemia 5
glutamate 4, 46
glutamine 8
glycopyrrolate 68
grimacing reflex 137f
Guillain-Barré syndrome 68

Harris-Benedict formulas 110–11
headache, orthostatic 39, 40
heart. *See* cardiac function
hemispheric lesions 130, 134, 135, 138, 141, 142
hemorrhage
  gastrointestinal 112–13, 114
  intracranial. *See* intracranial hemorrhage
heparin 37
hepatic failure 7–8
Heschl's gyrus 50f
histamine 46
histamine-2 receptor antagonists 109, 112
Horner's syndrome 134
hydralazine 83
hydrocephalus 29, 34–38, 36f, 39f, 40, 143
hydrocortisone 87
hypercapnia/hypercarbia 19, 31, 62
hyperemia 39
hypermetabolism 110
hyperosmolar therapy 20, 22–23, 23f, 25–26, 31
hypertension, intracranial. *See* intracranial pressure
hypertension, vascular 77, 80
  management 81–83, 86–87
hypertonic saline 23, 25–26
hyperventilation 62
  central neurogenic 65
  in raised ICP 20, 22, 26
hypoglycemia 5
hypotension, intracranial 38–40
hypotension, vascular 12–13, 31, 77
  management 83–85, 87–88
hypothalamus 134
  anterior 96
  posterior 45, 47
hypothermia, therapeutic 26

hypoventilation syndrome 65
hypoxemia 3, 12–13, 62, 63, 67

ICP. *See* intracranial pressure
ileus 106, 108–9, 113–14
immune suppression 110
incontinence, urinary 120–22
infections
  CNS 7
  septic shock 85, 87
  urinary tract 123, 124
inflammation 4, 6–7
inotropic effect 78, 85, 93
intestinal motility 105, 106, 108–9, 113–14
intracranial hemorrhage 12, 142
  subarachnoid 35, 86, 96, 99, 142
  subdural hematoma 6, 38, 40
  after ventriculostomy 37
intracranial hypotension 38–40
intracranial pressure (ICP) 17–27
  management 17, 22–26, 23f, 27
  monitoring 21–22, 21f, 24, 25, 27
  pathophysiology 18–22, 19f, 34, 35, 81, 91
intubation 67, 70
invasive mechanical ventilation 69–75, 69f
ischemia
  cardiac 82
  cerebral 3–4, 11, 35, 135

kidney failure 25

labetalol 81, 86, 100
lactate to pyruvate ratio 11
light reflex 133–34, 136, 137f
liver failure 7–8
localization of lesions 35, 129–43
locus coeruleus 46
lorazepam 68
losartan 82
lumbar drains
  in aortic aneurysm repair 40–41
  in hydrocephalus 36f, 37–38

magnetic resonance imaging (MRI)
  hydrocephalus 35
  intracranial hypotension 38, 40
  unconscious patients (fMRI) 43, 48–51, 49f, 50f, 53
malnutrition 111
management 12–13
  breathing difficulties 65, 67–74, 69f
  cardiac arrhythmias 97, 99–100
  CSF leaks 38
  gastric stress ulcers 112–13
  gastrointestinal motility disorders 109, 113–14
  hydrocephalus 36–38, 36f, 39f, 40
  hypertension 81–83, 85–86
  hypotension 83–85, 87–88

  nutrition 110–11
  raised ICP 17, 22–26, 23f, 27
  unconsciousness 46, 53–54
  urological disorders 122–25
mannitol 23, 23f, 25, 31
MCS (minimally conscious state) 43, 49, 50–51, 53, 54
mechanical ventilation 65, 67–74, 69f
medulla oblongata 60, 64, 79, 131, 134
meperidine 26
mesencephalon (midbrain) 35, 131, 134, 136, 141, 143
metabolism 1, 11, 14, 48, 110
methylnaltrexone 114
methylphenidate 54
metoclopramide 109, 114
metoprolol 81, 100
micronutrients 110
micturition 117–20, 118f
midbrain (mesencephalon) 35, 131, 134, 136, 141, 143
milrinone 84, 85
minimally conscious state (MCS) 43, 49, 50–51, 53, 54
minute ventilation 70, 71
miosis 133–34, 136
monitoring of patients 9–12
  EEG 9, 10, 11, 26, 51
  ICP 21–22, 21f, 24, 25, 27
Monro-Kellie doctrine 18, 39
motilin 108
motility drugs 109, 113–14
motor neuron disease 139
multiple sclerosis 65, 121
multisystem atrophy 121
muscles, neurological tests 138, 139
muscular dystrophy 98
myasthenia gravis 68, 98
myocarditis 98
myotonic dystrophy 98

naloxone 109
nasal cannulation 66–7
necrosis
  myocardial 93, 94f, 95
  neural 3, 5
neostigmine 68, 114
neuroendocrine agents
  cardiac 95
  gastrointestinal 106–8
neurogenic bladder 117, 120–26
neuroimaging 12, 141
  hydrocephalus 35
  intracranial hypotension 38, 40
  in unconscious patients 43, 48–51, 49f, 50f, 53
neurologic examination 52, 129–43, 137f
neurotoxins 3, 7–8

neurotransmitters
  blood pressure 78, 83, 84, 85, 87
  cardiac function 91, 93,
  consciousness 46–47
  gastrointestinal function 106
  ischemia 4
nicardipine 86
nizatidine 109
NMDA receptors 4
no-reflow phenomenon 20
noninvasive mechanical ventilation 68
norepinephrine (noradrenaline)
  blood pressure 78, 83, 84, 85, 87
  cardiac function 91, 93, 95
  gastrointestinal function 106
nucleus tractus solitarius 60, 79, 93–94, 96
nutrition 109–11

obese patients 111
occipital lobe lesions 130, 132
oculovestibular reflex 135, 136–37, 137f
Ogilvie syndrome 113–14
Ondine's curse 65
ophthalmologic examinations 35, 132–35, 137f
  in comatose patients 52, 134, 136, 141–42
opioid antagonists 109, 114
opioids
  gastrointestinal side-effects 108, 109, 113
  respiratory depression 64, 65
  in sedated patients 26
oropharyngeal weakness 66
orthostatic headache 39, 40
osmolality 25, 31
osmotic diuretics 20, 22–23, 23f, 25, 31
overactive bladder 120, 121, 122, 124
oxygen
  brain tissue oximetry 11
  cerebral blood flow 20, 81
  fMRI 48
  hypoxemia 3, 12–13, 62, 63, 67
  respiratory control 61–63, 62f, 72
  therapy 67

pain perception in MCS 51
paraplegia 138–39
parasympathetic nervous system
  bladder function 118–20, 118f, 119f
  blood pressure 22, 79, 79f
  cardiac function 92, 92f, 93, 96
  gastrointestinal function 106, 107f
  pupil size 133, 133f
parenteral nutrition 109
parietal lobe lesions 130
Parinaud's syndrome 35
Parkinson's disease 121
paroxysmal sympathetic hyperactivity syndrome 82, 86–87
pathophysiology of acute brain injury 1–9, 2f, 14

peak airway pressure 69, 71
PEEP (positive end expiratory pressure) 68, 71, 73
pentobarbital 26
peptide YY 108
peripherally inserted central catheters (PICC lines) 25, 99
peristalsis 106
persistent vegetative state (PVS) 43, 47, 54
  diagnosis 49, 50, 51, 52–53, 136
PET (positron emission tomography) 48
pethidine (meperidine) 26
phenylephrine 83, 84, 84, 87
phlebitis 25
phrenic nerve 63, 66
pinprick testing, 138, 139
pons
  breathing 60, 61, 64, 65
  localization of lesions 131, 133, 134, 136, 143
  pontine micturition center 117–18
positioning the patient 25, 32, 68
positive end expiratory pressure (PEEP) 68, 71, 73
positron emission tomography (PET) 48
posterior circulation syndromes 38–40, 132
posture 25, 32, 68
pre-Bötzinger complex 60
precuneus 48, 50
prefrontal cortex 49, 118
pressure reactivity index (PRx) 22
pressure support 69f
pressure/volume curve in ICP 18–20, 19f, 21, 24
propofol 26, 99
prostate surgery 121
proton pump inhibitors (PPIs) 113
pupil size 35, 132–34, 133f, 136, 141
PVS (persistent vegetative state) 43, 47, 54
  diagnosis 49, 50, 51, 52–53, 136
pyruvate (lactate to pyruvate ratio) 11

QT interval 98, 99

radiography. See X-rays
ranitidine 109
RAP index 21
reflexes, testing 133–34, 135, 136–37, 137f
renal failure 25
respiratory failure 59, 63–65
  See also breathing
reticular alerting system 45, 46

sacral neuromodulation 125
sacral sparing 139
saddle anesthesia 139
SAH (subarachnoid hemorrhage) 35, 86, 96, 99, 142
saline solutions, hypertonic 23, 25–26
secondary mechanisms of brain injury 6, 8–9, 8f
  prevention 12–13
sedation 13, 26, 52, 99

seizures 7, 10, 98, 134
sensory testing 138, 139–40
septic shock 85, 87
serotonin 46
shock, management of hypotension 83–85, 87–88
shortness of breath. *See* dyspnea
sinoatrial (SA) node 92, 93
skull 6, 18
sleep apnea 64, 65
sodium ions 4, 31
sodium nitroprusside 82
speech abnormalities 141
spinal cord injury
 in aortic aneurysm surgery 40–41
 autonomic dysreflexia 86–87
 breathing and 66
 localization 138–40, 140f, 141
 urogenital system, 120, 121–22, 124, 125
spinal shock 84, 121, 139
spirometry 66
splanchnic nerves 106, 108
spreading depression/depolarization 11
starvation 110
stomach 105
 hemorrhage 112–13, 114
 motility 106, 108–9, 113–14
 stress ulcers 108, 112–13
stress-induced cardiomyopathy 91, 94–95, 97–98
 EKG abnormalities 98–99
stroke 40, 64, 65, 101, 120, 132
 ischemia 3–4
stupor 35
subarachnoid hemorrhage (SAH) 35, 86, 96, 99, 142
subdural hematoma 6, 38, 40
sympathetic nervous system
 bladder function 118–20, 118f, 119f
 blood pressure 78–79, 79f, 86–87
 cardiac function 92–94, 92f, 96
 gastrointestinal function 106, 107f, 108, 112
 pupil size 133, 133f
synchronized intermittent mandatory ventilation (SIMV) 69f, 69, 72

tachycardia 83, 83, 96, 99, 100
TBI. *See* traumatic brain injury
temporal lobe lesions 130
tetraplegia 138–39
thalamus
 consciousness/unconsciousness 45, 46, 47, 135–36, 141
 localization of lesions to 132, 134, 143
therapeutic hypothermia 26
thiamine 111
thiopental 25
thoracoabdominal aortic aneurysm 40–41
thrombolysis 37
tidal volume 70, 71

tolterodine 124
tracheostomy 13, 73
transcranial magnetic stimulation 51
transplantation protocols 87
traumatic brain injury (TBI) 5–6
 coma 47, 52–53
 deterioration 142
 hyperventilation 65
 ICP monitoring 25
treatment. *See* management
tumors 35, 65

ulcers, gastric 108, 112–13
unconsciousness 43–54
 examination 51–53, 134, 135–37, 137f, 138, 141–42
 management 46, 53–54
 neuroanatomy and neurophysiology 44–48, 45f
 neuroimaging 43, 48–51, 49f, 50f, 52
urinary retention 120, 123, 124
urinary system 117–26
 anatomy and physiology 117–20, 118f, 119f
 neurological disorders 120–26
urinary tract infections 123, 124

vagus nerve
 cardiovascular function 22, 93
 gastrointestinal function 106
vascular tone 78–80
 ICP and 19, 20, 25, 31, 81
vasodilatory shock 87
vasogenic edema 6, 9, 80
vasopressin 84, 85, 87, 88, 97
Vaughan Williams classification 100
venous system 30–31, 30f, 34
ventilation, mechanical 65, 67–74, 69f
ventral respiratory group (VRG) 60
ventricular function/arrhythmia 93, 96, 99, 100
ventriculoperitoneal CSF shunts 32, 37, 38, 39f
ventriculostomy 24, 36–37, 36f, 38, 40
vital capacity 66
vomiting 105

wakefulness. *See* consciousness
Wallerian degeneration 5–6
warfarin 37
watershed areas 3–4
weakness, examination 132, 137–40
weaning from mechanical ventilation 73
Wernicke-Korsakoff syndrome 111
white matter 5–6, 12, 135
 demyelination 6–7, 8

X-rays
 dyspnea 66
 ventriculoperitoneal shunts 39f

zolpidem 46, 54